Coping with Chronic Pain

A Guide to Patient Self-Management

Richard W. Hanson

Kenneth E. Gerber

The Guilford Press
New York   London

© 1990 The Guilford Press
A Division of Guilford Publications, Inc.
72 Spring Street, New York, NY· 10012

Printed in the United States of America

This book is printed on acid-free paper.

Last digit is print number: 9 8 7 6 5 4 3 2

Library of Congress Cataloging-in-Publication Data

Hanson, Richard W., 1944–
    Coping with chronic pain: a guide to patient self-management /
Richard W. Hanson, Kenneth E. Gerber.
        p.   cm.
    Includes bibliographical references.
    ISBN 0-89862-396-0   ISBN 0-89862-549-1 (pbk.)
    1. Intractable pain. 2. Self-care, Health.   I. Gerber, Kenneth
E.   II. Title.
    [DNLM: 1. Adaptation, Psychological. 2. Chronic Disease.
3. Pain–prevention & control. 4. Self Care—methods. WL 704
H251c]
    RB127.H37   1990
    616'.0472—dc20
    DNLM/DLC   89-17204
    for Library of Congress   CIP

Foreword

The past two decades have witnessed an explosion of interest in and research on chronic pain. Exciting advances have been made in both the basic scientific understanding of the mechanisms underlying nociception and in the development of innovative therapeutic interventions. That is the good news. This optimistic pronouncement might lead to a belief that the research has led to or is on the verge of totally eliminating human suffering. Unfortunately, despite advances in our understanding of the neurochemistry and basic physiology subserving nociception, as well as of surgical and pharmacological advances, satisfactory elimination of pain remains elusive. If epidemiological research is any indication, the incidence of chronic pain is escalating rather than abating—example, during the 20-year period from 1957 to 1976, social security disability awards increased by 300%, with disability for back pain increasing alone by 2700%!

The reader might ask how it is possible that the accretion of knowledge of basic physical mechanisms did not produce adequate "cures" for pain. The response is that with the advances in knowledge of physiology there has been a simultaneous appreciation of the complexity of chronic pain, especially the important modulating role of psychological variables. Simply administering advanced surgical techniques or potent analgesic agents has not resulted in dramatic reductions in complaints of persistent pain. Cognitive, affective, and behavioral factors have all been demonstrated to play a role in perception and behavioral response to chronic pain. Thus, it is no longer possible to view pain as a purely sensory phenomenon but rather as a complex perceptual experience. Cognitive appraisals of nociceptive stimuli based on prior learning history, the meaning of the context in which nociceptive stimuli are perceived, and evaluation of resources for controlling noxious sensory input (both medical and personal) all have a direct effect on emotional state. Moreover, emotional factors influence physiological parameters, behavioral responses, and appraisal processes. And, environmental reinforcement contingencies influence subsequent thoughts and feelings as well as behavior.

With increased knowledge has come a greater appreciation of the reciprocal interactions between physical perturbations and psychological parameters. This is especially the case when it is acknowledged that by virtue of definition *chronic* pain extends over time. For example, it is not unusual for the mean duration of pain reported in pain-clinic samples to exceed 7 years. When we take a longitudinal perspective, it becomes quite obvious that to treat chronic pain successfully, we must consider not only physical pathology but the myriad of psychosocial and behavioral factors that influence the responses of chronic-pain sufferers. It is this longitudinal view that underscores the complexity of chronic pain.

To acknowledge the chronic aspect of pain requires that we go beyond simple reliance on biomedical models, which have greater relevance in discussion and treatment of acute-pain states (a caveat—cognitive, affective, and behavioral factors have been shown to play important roles in acute pain, as well as chronic pain). When a disease or result of an injury persists over time, it impacts on all areas of functioning—familial, economic, vocational, social, as well as physical. The physical contributors (nociceptive sensory stimuli) to pain perception may have influenced the initial perceptual experience, but over time, these factors are modulated by what patients think, feel, and the environmental response.

What happens when the symptoms do not remit? Referrals for medical consultations, rounds of more sophisticated diagnostic tests, and perhaps surgery, accompanied by greater fear, symptom preoccupation, reduced activity and physical deconditioning, family distress, withdrawal from usual activities, depression, physiological arousal, and potential legal adversarial issues related to disability compensation are all set in motion. Failure to recover may lead to questions being raised as to the veracity of the complaints and questions of secondary gains if not to concerns about downright malingering which in turn contribute to psychological distress and behavioral responses. Maladaptive cognitive expectations and appraisals regarding the health care system and legal system, social support, and the future may further facilitate feelings of psychological distress and lead to still greater inactivity. Fear of greater injury or further degeneration may reduce an ever widening range of activities. Inactivity and increased use of narcotic medication will alter sleep patterns, inducing lethargy and failure of usual coping strategies. Psychological distress may increase muscle tension and further exacerbate pain. Secondary iatrogenic (negative consequences of medical treatment) and jurisogenic (negative consequences of the legal system) factors may also contribute to a worsening situation. In short, the chronic-pain sufferer enters a vicious, accelerating downward spiral which extends over time and impacts not only on the identified patient but on his or her entire family.

The all-to-familiar portrait sketched above has resulted in the development of specialty clinics designed to treat the health care system failures— chronic-pain patients. Treatment of chronic pain can be viewed as a growth industry. It has been estimated that over 2000 pain treatment facilities exist in the United States alone. Despite the large number of pain clinics, only a score of these programs have been described in the literature. All too often all we know about their methods is confined to a handful of descriptive paragraphs in journal articles reporting on treatment outcome. The discussion sections of these articles typically describe the clinical efficacy of the methods used; however, it is difficult for the reader to determine what was actually included within the treatment regimen. Vague mention of "cognitive–behavioral," "operant," and "multidisciplinary" orientations are presented as descriptive; however, there is no agreement as to what these terms connote in actual practice. This relative neglect tends to promote a "treatment uniformity," whereby it is assumed that all "operant treatments," for example, are equivalent. There have been only a handful of books that have provided detail sufficient to enable the practicing clinician to adopt the therapeutic strategy and actually make use of the recommended tactics.

In this volume, Hanson and Gerber provide a detailed description of a self-management approach to the treatment of patients with recalcitrant chronic pain. They base their conceptualization on a biopsychosocial model in contrast to the more conventional biomedical model. The self-control conceptualization adopted by the authors takes a central, systems, chronic-illness view that can be contrasted with a peripheral, reductionistic, acute-disease view. They emphasize the role of cognitive and behavioral factors in *understanding* the plight of the chronic-pain sufferer.

Strategically, the authors' self-management perspective focuses on: health care provider–patient collaboration, treatment flexibility and customization of treatment techniques to meet the needs of individual patients, and emphasis on self-acceptance, coping versus cure, resourcefulness versus helplessness, and activity versus passivity. The tactics described are quite variable, and include physical activity enhancement and patterning, education in the use of problem solving, cognitive and behavioral coping skills, assertion, and relaxation training. The authors caution against the rigidity of promoting specific techniques, and thereby trying to fit square pegs into round holes—the "patient uniformity myth." They eschew the hammer–nail approach where all patients are treated the same because only one set of techniques is deemed by the therapist to be the "correct one," a panacea for all, and where the tendency is to view the treatment as a success but the patient as the cause of failure when outcome does not meet the clinician's expectations.

A major advantage of this book is the authors' attention to the importance of the theoretical rationale of the treatment. They emphasize that the self-management model should pervade all facets of the treatment program and the need for this common perspective to be adhered to by all clinical team members.

The conceptual model or perspective that one holds about chronic pain will influence the way patients are thought about, the assessment methods used, the treatment modalities employed, and the manner in which treatment is conducted. All to often the pain treatment literature is eclectic (multidisciplinary) with more attention given to tactics (what) and strategy (how) at the expense of rationale (why). In this volume, the authors balance the philosophical underpinnings of the self-management approach with specific treatment strategies and tactics making judicious use of clinical-case vignettes to illustrate their points. The "nonspecifics" of their approach are given equal attention to the treatment techniques, and the authors take care to describe the rationale for the selection and methods of use of all therapeutic modalities.

Hanson and Gerber broach a number of clinically "nociceptive" topics that rarely are mentioned in discussions of various pain-treatment modalities; for example, preparation for treatment, presenting the need to eliminate use of narcotics, identification of patients who are *not* likely to benefit from the clinician's preferred approach and how these non-candidates should be treated, how patient resistance should be addressed, what should be done with disruptive patients, and how adherence, maintenance, and generalization should be incorporated within the treatment plan.

The authors nicely interweave relevant research within the fabric of their approach. Yet they do not let themselves be held hostage to available research literature. There are many gaps in our understanding of chronic pain and chronic-pain patients and the authors are willing to go with clinical experience when data are unavailable.

This concise and well-written volume should be read by all health care professionals, especially pain-management teams who treat chronic-pain patients, regardless of theoretical orientation or professional training. The self-management perspective can be readily applied regardless of the clinician's training or preferred treatment modalities. Moreover, the strategies and tactics can supplement clinician's therapeutic armamentariums.

The authors' emphasis on the patient's own perspective on the problems and treatments offered should sensitize health care providers, of all persuasions, to the central position of the target of their efforts. It is all too easy to lose sight of the individual patient in our zeal for our preferred model and approaches. Failure to consider the relevant patient characteristics and the patient's perspective will inevitably contribute to therapeutic failure, resistance, nonadherence, and relapse, and thereby clinician frustration. It is all too easy for clinicians to blame failure on patients without considering their own contributions to treatment outcome.

I urge the reader to examine his or her conceptualizations, strategies, and tactics in light of those presented here. The success of this volume will depend upon whether reading it changes health care providers' thinking about chronic-pain patients and perhaps more importantly whether their behavior changes. The outcome of such modifications should lead to more effective treatment of this most challenging population.

Dennis C. Turk
University of Pittsburgh School of Medicine

Contents

CHAPTER 1

Introduction

In recent years both social scientists and health care professionals have been working toward the development of a new theoretical perspective on health and illness. Conceptions of health and illness continuously change as they reflect social, technological, and philosophical trends (Stone, 1979). The lack of a consensus regarding a proper definition of health contributes significantly to difficult clinical situations that we read about every day in both professional health journals and the daily newspaper. Such issues as how to best use innovative new medical technologies, disagreement over appropriate medical and psychosocial criteria for maintaining a terminally ill patient's life, and how to distribute health-care dollars among the diverse needs of the rapidly increasing population of elderly and chronically ill individuals are but a few of these dilemmas for which there are no clear solutions. These controversies reflect the fact that technological advances in medicine have far surpassed our ability to achieve agreement on these more abstract, value-laden issues related to the provision of medical care.

The development of alternative models of health and illness is perhaps nowhere better illustrated than in the area that comprises the subject of this book, chronic pain. The medical and psychological communities, both scientific and clinical, have long debated about the characteristics, development, and treatment of pain. As with conceptualizations of health and illness in general, our understanding of pain has reflected the dominant philosophical paradigms of each era. Aristotle's notion of pain as an emotion and not a fundamentally physical phenomenon mirrored Greek thought concerning the relationship between mind and body. In the Middle Ages, pain was closely tied to religious thought and was viewed as punishment for sin, a view that rejected the body as the true source of pain. The historical period of the Enlightenment, with its emphasis on rationality, the scientific method, and its faith in human progress through technology, led to a radically different view of pain. Illich (1976) traces this scientific perspective through the writings of Descartes who, in emphasizing the separation of mind and body, described pain as purely a functional mechanism that signaled bodily damage.

Illich describes the influence of Cartesian philosophy on the beginning of medical technology aimed at "killing pain." As pain came to be viewed as something that merely interfered with the efficiency of the human machine, inevitably the attitude would develop that pain could be eliminated through rationally developed, mechanistic techniques. Pain was increasingly understood as something to be avoided at all costs, in contrast to earlier views that depicted pain as having significant spiritual and emotional meaning. The individual who suffered from pain was a passive victim whose pain could be taken away by experts. The elimination of pain became the central focus of those interested in the topic, and reflection on the nontechnical issues related to pain was discouraged.

This evolving view of pain paralleled theoretical and clinical developments throughout science and medicine. More and more, medicine became dominated by a mechanistic view of the body and disease. American medicine has become perhaps the most mechanistic in orientation of all Western societies (Payer, 1988). American medicine is particularly aggressive in treating disease. Unlike Europeans, Americans tend to view themselves as naturally healthy. They believe disease and pain to be externally caused nuisances that science and technology are responsible for eliminating. Other cultural factors reinforce this perspective. For example, the system of financial reimbursement for medical services in America seems to have built-in incentives for the excessive use of medical procedures in both evaluation and treatment. Later in this book, we describe in more detail the implications of these traditional theories of disease and pain as a way of introducing an alternative biopsychosocial model. Before exploring these models in depth, we consider the problem of chronic pain in general and one particularly common type of chronic-pain condition, low back pain.

THE PROBLEM OF CHRONIC PAIN

Researchers from diverse disciplines have identified pain, especially chronic pain, as a critical national problem. In their review of the epidemiology of pain, Osterweis, Kleinman, and Mechanic (1987) note that approximately 10% of all individuals in the United States have pain conditions on more than 100 days per year, including 7 million individuals who suffer from low back pain at any one time. The National Center for Health Statistics found over a recent 3-year period that there were 70 million physician visits in which pain was the primary complaint; of these, 10 million were for back pain. Pain-related visits represent the vast majority of all appointments with physicians. These staggering numbers translate into over 4 billion lost work days for pain conditions, one third of which are for low back pain (Osterweis et al., 1987). Chronic-pain conditions such as arthritis and migraine headaches affect tens of millions of people. As an example of the financial burden of such conditions in the United States, it has been noted that low back pain alone costs at least 16 billion dollars per year (Frymoyer, 1988). Approximately one-third of this amount is for medical costs, and the remaining two-thirds are for compensation.

Recently, the Nuprin Pain Report, conducted by the Louis Harris Polling Associates (Taylor & Curran, 1985), studied the epidemiology of pain conditions in the United States. The major pain conditions identified in the survey were headache, backache, muscle and joint pain, stomach pain, menstrual cycle pain, and dental pain. These accounted for 98% of all patient complaints. Back pain, joint pain, and headache occurred in about one of seven people. Chronic muscle pain was found in 1 of 10 people, and other types of chronic pain affected 1 of 20 individuals. The Nuprin study found that over 14% of all Americans missed at least 1 day of work per year because of pain. The percentage of those reporting pain decreased with education level and increased with age. Other studies have concluded that new pain cases are highest in younger patients, and chronic pain is more common in older individuals, especially women (Osterweis et al., 1987). Low occupational status correlates with greater complaints of pain. This finding could be the result of the less prestigious occupations often being more physically demanding and having a greater likelihood of physical damage. Among the clearest findings of the Nuprin survey is the predominance of back pain as the single most prevalent source of pain, especially chronic pain. We now examine the phenomenon of low back pain to illustrate the difficulties associated with the treatment of chronic-pain conditions.

LOW BACK PAIN

As the Nuprin study revealed, low back pain is among the most common pain complaints for which patients visit their physician. It is the most common cause of work days missed because of disability related to pain. Harris and associates found that 14% of the adult population have serious chronic back pain conditions, and about the same percentage suffer less severe back pain that is still significant enough to interfere with daily work or routine. Such findings of the incidence of chronic back pain have generally been replicated in investigations in other Western countries such as Sweden and Denmark (Osterweis et al., 1987). Low back pain is the major cause of morbidity and disability in people between the ages of 18 and 44, the most active, productive work years.

Occasional episodes of low back pain are very common. Estimates of lifetime prevalence for sufferers range from 60% to 90% (Frymoyer, 1988). The vast majority of these episodes are time-limited with 80-90% resolving within 6 weeks (Waddell, 1987). Although some individuals report recurring episodes of low back pain, most do not bother to seek medical treatment. Research studies indicate that a small percentage of the total of all individuals who suffer from occasional low back pain develop chronic, persistent back pain. A large-scale Canadian study of patients with work-related back pain found that 7% developed into chronic conditions (Spitzer & Quebec Task Force on Spinal Disorders, 1987). According to Frymoyer (1988), the 5% of individuals who have persisting pain symptoms beyond 3 months account for 85% of the costs in terms of compensation and loss of work resulting from low back pain. Why some people develop chronic low back pain conditions and others do not is unknown at this time.

Diagnosis of Low Back Pain

Low back pain has perplexed physicians because of the difficulty in arriving at a definitive diagnosis. Numerous diagnostic terms are found in the literature such as lumbar strain or lumbar sprain, lumbago, sciatica, diskal hernia, diskopathy, facet syndrome, lumbar myositis, ligamentitis, minor intervertebral displacement, dysfunction of the intervertebral joint, fibromyositis, fibrositis, fasciitis, myofasciitis, articular hypomobility and hypermobility, diskarthrosis, etc. (Spitzer & Quebec Task Force, 1987). Some of these labels assume the presence of structural problems involving the spine, whereas others assume that the source of pain is found in the soft tissues (i.e., muscles, fascia, ligaments).

Although x-ray abnormalities are not uncommon in back pain patients, these findings do not usually correlate in any consistent way with patient complaints. For example, it is known that disk degeneration increases with age even though low back pain and disability do not (Waddell, 1987). Those who emphasize soft tissue problems must rely more on physical examination rather than imaging procedures such as x rays, CAT scans, and magnetic resonance imaging (MRI). This has also led to a confusing array of diagnoses such as myofascial pain, fibromyalgia, fibrositis, and so forth, which are not fully accepted in the medical community (Osterweis et al., 1987). Nevertheless, a recent survey of physicians specializing in pain indicated that physical examination procedures such as neurological examination, observation of gait and posture, assessment of spinal mobility, examination of muscular function, examination of soft tissues, and assessment of mobility of weight-bearing joints are preferred over other technological procedures (Rudy, Turk, & Brena, 1988). Part of the diagnostic dilemma results from the fact that physicians, when conducting the physical exam, must always rely to some extent on patients' reports of pain and associated pain/disability behaviors that are subject to considerable influence by psychosocial factors. Thus, the failure to distinguish among pain associated with observable injury or disease, learned pain behavior, and the suffering/distress component of pain has lead to considerable diagnostic confusion (Fordyce, 1988; Loeser, 1982; Waddell, 1987).

Medical and Surgical Treatment

Numerous treatment approaches have been used for low back pain including those that comprise the following list: acupuncture, back schools, bed rest, biofeedback, chemonucleolysis, cryotherapy, denervation, diskectomy, electroanalgesia, exercises in a specialized center, functional training, home exercises, intervention of occupational aspects, laminectomy, laminotomy, local medication, manipulation, massage, medication, mobilization, pain clinic treatment, postural information, psychopharmacology, psychotherapy, return to work, spinal arthrodesis, spinal orthosis, spinal support, strengthening exercises, stretching exercises, systemic medication, thermotherapy, traction, and work cessation (Spitzer & Quebec Task Force, 1987).

Considerable attention has been given to surgical interventions, since they often appear to be the most direct means of correcting the presumed cause of back pain. Surgeons can operate on presumed structural problems in the spine (e.g., bulging or protruding disks) even though the relationship between those structural problems and pain complaints/disability is low. Although surgery may be necessary for cases of acute low back pain when certain neurological findings are present, it is often unsuccessful among those who have suffered low back pain for any length of time. In fact, it has been suggested that successful disk surgery applies to only about 1% of patients with low back disorders (Waddell, 1987). Nevertheless, low back surgery is being performed in this country at an increasing rate. In 1986, about 400,000 surgeries for lumbar disk disease were done. Most studies report that the majority of persons who undergo such surgery are no better off in the long run than those who were treated

conservatively. Specifically, patients who have surgery for these conditions at 4 and 10 years follow-up, compared to equivalent groups who
did not have surgery, have the same functional and symptomatic characteristics (Weber, 1983). Additionally, further back surgeries on the same
individual for whom the first surgery failed also usually fail, and at
increasingly higher rates. Repeat back surgery fails at a rate twice that of
first-time surgery. A third surgery is 10 times more likely to fail than a
second surgery. Failure in such cases is usually defined as failure to relieve
pain, which, it must be remembered, is the patient's main complaint.
Thus, low back surgery may be successful from a strictly technical
perspective (i.e., repair of a herniated disk) but not from the patient's
perspective (i.e., pain relief).

Waddell and his colleagues (Waddell, Kummel, Lotto, Graham,
Hall, & McCulloch, 1979; Waddell, McCulloch, Kummel, & Venner,
1980), in noting the poor prospect for successful repeat surgery with these
patients, suggest that few of the potential cases should actually have had
surgery in the first place. Waddell et al. (1980) recommend that greater
attention be given to an examination of nonorganic signs and psychological factors, so that unnecessary surgery is avoided. In support of this
recommendation, Gore, Sepic, Gardner, and Murray (1987), in a study of
205 patients with chronic upper back and neck pain, found that it was not
possible to predict which medical treatment would be most appropriate
for a specific patient based on presenting physical symptoms or x-ray
findings only. The presence or absence of pain 10 years after the original
symptoms was found unrelated to even the most fundamental physical
measures including degenerative or sclerotic changes in the cervical spine.

A significant amount of research conducted by surgeons has focused
on identifying relevant physical and psychosocial characteristics of the
low back pain syndrome. For example, Long, Filtzer, BenDebba, and
Hendler (1988) examined the clinical features of 78 patients who had
undergone unsuccessful back surgery. Sophisticated diagnostic test (e.g.,
computerized tomography) results were reviewed by a neurosurgeon and
orthopedist for each of the study participants. It was found that 16 of the
patients had no physical abnormalities that could explain their back pain,
and 13 had documented physical abnormalities that were insufficient to
explain their condition. Of the 78 patients in the study, 27 had physical
complications directly related to previous back surgery. Fifty-two of the
patients were judged to have a physical condition that did not warrant
surgery. Almost 75% of these patients needed back surgery to correct the
effects of previous surgery. The authors conclude that many patients
present themselves to surgeons with persistent pain complaints for which
there is little physical evidence. These patients often undergo surgery that

fails, resulting in greater physical damage, increased pain, and narcotic addiction. Long et al. (1988) suggest that psychological evaluation might be able to screen out those back-pain patients unlikely to be helped by surgery.

Alternative Models of Low Back Pain

It has been noted that many patients' chronic back pain complaints and disability appear out of proportion to any observable physical abnormalities. This can lead the clinician to assume that the patient's pain is psychologically caused or functional in origin. Most research, however, does not support a clear dichotomy between functional and organic pain. Keel (1984) reviewed 18 research studies that focused on the identification of criteria differentiating organic from functional pain in back-pain patients. He found that only two of the studies concluded that such a differentiation was possible. Importantly, little evidence could be found that individuals with low back pain of unknown physical origin necessarily had premorbid psychological disturbance. Keel's review supports the notion that back pain is often difficult to diagnose and is probably best understood from a biopsychosocial, rather than an exclusively medical, perspective.

Waddell and his colleagues have written extensively about the development of alternative models of low back pain that incorporate the evidence from studies such as those discussed above (Waddell, 1987; Waddell, Morris, DiPaola, Bircher, & Finlayson, 1986). They note that surgical and other medical treatment decisions involving low-back-pain patients are too often made on the basis of the perceived suffering and disability of the patient rather than the actual physical findings (Waddell, 1987). In an extensive review of the treatment outcome data, he concludes that there is no evidence that any treatment for low back pain is better than "a combination of the natural history and the placebo effect" (Waddell, 1987, p. 636). Patients' pain complaints seem to have more to do with feelings of distress than purely physical sensations. As such, individuals may have minimal or no physical findings related to their pain even though they present high distress. These patients present the most difficult management problems for health care providers.

Chronic-pain patients, particularly those with back pain, represent a significant challenge to the health care system both in terms of financial cost and as a reminder of the need to develop more effective therapeutic strategies for pain relief. Spitzer and his Quebec Task Force (1987) concluded from their study that the management of the high-demand chronic-pain patient, including the identification of proper diagnostic and prognostic modalities, should be the most critical research priority of the pain specialist. As is discussed in the next chapter, this task can be facilitated by the adoption of a broader conceptual framework regarding pain. Along with others, we refer to such a perspective as the biopsychosocial model.

THE CHRONIC-PAIN SYNDROME

Health care professionals are becoming increasingly aware of the significant distinction between acute and chronic pain. The vast majority of pain episodes are acute. Such pain occurrences are temporary and resolve either on their own or after appropriate medical treatment. Nevertheless, some individuals develop chronic recurrent or persistent pain conditions. At least three subtypes of chronic pain can be distinguished. In some cases an ongoing disease process can be identified that results in persistent pain. Unfortunately, the particular disease does not resolve on its own and is not subject to curative medical treatment. Examples include various arthritic conditions, certain cancers, and chronic pancreatitis. This type of pain is similar to most cases of acute pain in that a peripheral source of nociception can be identified. Second are cases in which there is clear evidence of injury or presumed pathological processes that directly involve peripheral or central nerve structures. Causalgia, various neuralgias (e.g., postherpetic neuralgia, trigeminal neuralgia), postamputation pain, pain associated with spinal cord injury, malignancies affecting the nerves, and the thalamic pain syndrome are examples. The relationship between nerve damage and pain is not clearly understood, since some individuals with clear evidence of nerve damage report no pain, whereas others present severe, debilitating pain (Loeser, 1985). Finally, there are cases in which peripheral disease processes or nerve damage cannot be clearly identified. Many within this category originally had an acute pain condition that persisted beyond the expected disease course or healing processes. In such cases it is usually presumed that psychological factors play a predominant role in maintaining the person's pain.

Some individuals with chronic pain who present clear evidence of peripheral disease or nerve damage are able to cope successfully with their conditions and to minimize the disabling effects. These individuals may continue to be employed or be engaged in other forms of productive activity in spite of their chronic pain. Since they have been able to accept and adapt to their pain, they usually do not place repeated demands on the health care system to eliminate or significantly reduce their pain.

Others with chronic pain develop a number of unfortunate characteristics that can be referred to as the chronic-pain syndrome. This syndrome includes a number of behaviors and psychological characteristics that supersede the specific physical aspects of the pain condition. Those who have developed the chronic-pain syndrome may present several of the following features:

1. A history of repeated unsuccessful attempts to obtain medical or surgical relief for their pain problem.
2. The presentation of physical disability in excess of what may be expected or necessitated by the medical condition.
3. Repeated attempts to obtain financial compensation for the painful condition (e.g., lawsuits, worker's compensation, and other types of disability compensation).
4. Dependence on narcotic analgesics, anxiolytic or sedative medication, alcohol, or illicit drugs as a means of coping with pain.
5. Development of a variety of dysfunctional psychosocial symptoms including depression, sleep disturbance, conflicts with health care providers and family members, significant decrease in physical activity, loss of gratification from daily activities, preoccupation with pain and other somatic complaints, use of pain to control and manipulate other people or to avoid unwanted responsibilities and tasks, and so forth.

These characteristics may be present in varying degrees of intensity across chronic-pain patients. Some of these features are easily identified, whereas others are based more on social judgments of a particular individual. Those who present with this syndrome are most likely to be referred to specialty pain clinics.

This syndrome is sometimes referred to as the chronic intractable *benign* pain syndrome to distinguish it from chronic pain associated with cancer (Crue, 1983; Crue & Pinsky, 1984). The use of the word "benign" is unfortunate, since the syndrome is far from benign. Nevertheless, it is important to emphasize that the self-management principles and procedures described in this book were developed primarily for those whose pain is *not* directly associated with a neoplastic process. In particular, our strong opposition to the use of narcotic analgesics does not apply to those whose pain is caused by cancer. Such patients, especially those in the terminal phases of the disease, may require rational treatment with narcotic analgesics. In spite of this exception, we do believe that the biopsychosocial model applies to those with cancer pain and that such patients can benefit from many self-management approaches. We do not believe, however, that such patients are appropriate candidates for a comprehensive chronic-pain-management program described in the following chapters.

The evaluation and treatment of those with the chronic-pain syndrome from the traditional medical perspective produces multiple frustrations for both patient and health care provider. This book focuses on the description of an alternative biopsychosocial perspective on the evaluation and treatment of the chronic-pain patient. The theoretical basis of this model as well as its clinical implementation is emphasized. We describe the model's application with real patients without ignoring the significant complexities of individualized pain treatment. The authors' experience is based on the day-to-day operation of an outpatient pain clinic that evaluates 300 patients a year and intensively treats about 100 of these individuals within a 21-day inpatient program. We have worked with over 1,000 patients since the clinic's inception. Our self-management treatment model has evolved through stages of adaptaton as demanded by our clinical successes and failures. Although the well-known cognitive–behavioral model (Turk, Meichenbaum, & Genest, 1983) is the foundation of our approach, we have not always been satisfied with its rigid application to certain types of chronic-pain patients. Many of our pain patients are best approached from a flexible theoretical perspective that allows flexible treatment options. For example, we have found that in a significant percentage of patients, childhood and psychodynamic factors must also be addressed. Pain management in these cases cannot consist solely of structured instruction in pain-coping skills (e.g., relaxation training) but must be supplemented with longer-term psychotherapeutic approaches. Traditional psychotherapy can be an integral part of the self-management paradigm described in this book. Self-management is a philosophy of treatment that recognizes individual patient variability while appreciating the general similarities among individuals fitting the chronic-pain syndrome. We now briefly summarize those aspects of the self-management model covered in each chapter of this book.

OVERVIEW

Models of Pain

Chapter 2 begins with the assumption that everyone, including patients and health care professionals, possesses a conceptual model of pain. These models must be understood by the clinician, since they determine and thus also limit acceptable treatment options. Two particular models, the biomedical and biopsychosocial, are discussed in detail with respect to how they presume pain mechanisms to operate, how each views the phenomenology of the pain experience, and what are considered appropriate interventions. We describe the shortcomings of each model and emphasize situations in which each model is the preferred foundation for clinical intervention.

We believe that a biopsychosocial systems model provides the most comprehensive perspective for understanding the origin of all disease as well as generates a more flexible range of treatment options. Although biomedical treatment approaches are effective with many acute injuries and disease conditions, they tend to be less beneficial for many chronic conditions including persistent pain. Rather than focusing on repairing mechanical breakdowns in the body machine, the biopsychosocial model focuses more on the person with the chronic disease. How the person appraises, reacts to, and copes with the disease and its treatment are considered crucial issues in health care. The sociocultural context of the patient is also of vital importance.

In the case of those who present the chronic-pain syndrome, these personal perceptions, emotional reactions, coping behaviors, and social contextual factors become the primary targets of intervention. Repetitive efforts to repair the presumed mechanical cause of pain not only are seen as inadequate but can contribute in some cases to the development and maintenance of the chronic-pain syndrome. Self-management is offered as a major alternative to biomedical treatment. This approach requires that the patient assume much greater responsibility for the day-to-day management of the chronic condition.

Introduction to Self-Management Training

The third chapter describes the evaluation and preparation of chronic-pain patients for self-management training. The biopsychosocial model of pain is discussed in terms of reciprocal interactions among its components, including physical sensations, cognitive factors, emotional responses, overt behavior, and socioenvironmental features. The neurophysiological underpinnings of this model, including the gate-control theory, are briefly discussed. Self-management training primarily emphasizes change in cognition and behavior that, in turn, can alter each other component. Common self-management goals are summarized. Essential targets for change, based on treatment of affective disorders, include dysfunctional action tendencies, perceptions of uncontrollability and unpredictability, and self-focused attention.

Self-Management of Physical Activities

In Chapter 4 we discuss the critical issue of the physical activity of the chronic-pain patient. Whereas traditional medical approaches often discourage physical activity, self-management emphasizes appropriate types and amounts of activity. Since many chronic-pain patients experience the adverse consequences of physical disuse, an active physical reconditioning program must be instituted. Patients are taught to identify other factors that contribute to excess disability such as depression, fear, and avoidance and positive environmental consequences. Emphasis is placed on discovering true or necessary limitations, maintaining a balanced and modulated activity level within those limitations, and working toward healthy self-appraisals in spite of physical limitations.

Coping with Pain through Distraction

Chapter 5 discusses mechanisms of attentional refocusing and their use in coping with chronic pain. Additionally, we emphasize the importance of constructive activities (i.e., employment, volunteer work, personal and household responsibilities), hobbies and leisure-time pursuits, and social activities. Cognitive distraction techniques including relaxation and mental imagery are also described, particularly as to how they fit into overall self-management strategies. We address the many difficulties in the use of distraction with the chronic-pain patient and describe alternative ways of managing the patient resistant to the use of distraction.

Coping with Episodes of Intense Pain

Many of the chronic-pain patients we treat respond very positively to the self-management model, particularly in response to managing everyday levels of pain. Brief, intense pain episodes, however, often represent serious obstacles for patients. During such times, the patient is most likely to resort to dysfunctional coping behaviors (e.g., increased narcotic use, decreased activity levels). In Chapter 6, we emphasize a preventive approach to dealing with intense pain experiences. In addition, we describe steps for the patient to cope with intense pain in the most effective way possible without the use of narcotics.

Coping with Stress and Depression

In Chapter 7 we emphasize the importance of identifying sources of stress and interpersonal conflict in patients' lives and how these experiences relate to pain. Because the self-management model involves the individual assuming personal responsibility for managing stress and conflict as well as pain, we discuss the role of cognitive appraisal mechanisms with special emphasis on how cognitive distortions affect the individual's stress and pain levels. The well-researched relationship between depression and pain is discussed with particular reference to how certain cognitive and behavioral coping strategies may be used to reduce both conditions.

The Organization and Management of Chronic-Pain Programs

The structure and daily operation of pain programs must always reinforce the basic themes of the self-management model. In Chapter 8 we outline the alternative roles for the various staff members and describe the administrative organization of a multidisciplinary, comprehensive pain center. Optional clinic arrangements depending on staffing and budgetary constraints are discussed. Our emphasis is on describing, from the administrative point of view, how staff and patient difficulties are manageable in ways that reinforce the self-management philosophy.

Beyond Self-Management Training

We begin with the assertion that pain treatments (medical or psychological) can fail when clinicians fail to identify and address the most important factors (physical, psychological, or social) that are maintaining a particular patient's pain. Self-management training is no exception. This approach primarily aims at assisting those who have developed the chronic-pain syndrome to cope more effectively with the pain condition and its adverse consequences on their lives. It is less effective or relevant for those whose pain is secondary to other long-standing psychosocial problems. In some cases, chronic pain may be related to earlier emotionally painful life events, and for some, the chronic pain may serve as a dysfunctional solution to other, more prominent personal or family problems. In such cases, self-management training may need to be replaced by or supplemented with other psychotherapeutic approaches.

One of the most important goals in chronic-pain research and practice is to identify the most appropriate interventions for particular patients. In other words, treatment should match the needs of the patient rather than the patient be required to fit into a particular treatment approach. Four general treatment modalities are discussed that are appropriate for different categories of pain patients. These are the medical, self-management training, psychotherapeutic, and supportive counseling approaches.

Finally, it is important to recognize that a multidimensional biopsychosocial model applies to far more than those with chronic-pain conditions. Although we believe that this model applies to all types of illness, it is especially relevant for those conditions that reflect the limits of technological medicine. In particular, it is becoming increasingly apparent that this perspective has tremendous implications for the prevention and management of chronic disease conditions that are now the primary causes of mortality in this country. The most important of these implications is the necessity for all people to assume greater personal responsibility for managing their own health rather than placing all responsibility onto the medical care system.

CHAPTER 2

Models of Pain

To understand better the problem of chronic pain, it is important to recognize that nearly everyone who experiences it develops his or her own model of pain. Model in this context refers to a conceptual framework or paradigm that serves to guide one's understanding of the phenomenon of pain. A general model of pain can be considered to include two basic perspectives. First, it includes one's understanding and response to the subjective experience of pain. Second, it determines how one understands and reacts to pain in others. These models, or cognitive schemata, include assumptions regarding the cause of pain and what can be done about it. Models can vary on an explicit–implicit dimension. That is, some individuals consciously can recognize and clearly articulate their pain models (explicit), whereas for others, models remain at a more tacit or implicit level. Additionally, models can range between being highly differentiated and situation specific to being global and diffuse.

Pain models are very important for several reasons. First, pain models determine how scientists go about studying pain. The particular questions asked, research methods used, and the phenomena looked at are all determined by the scientist's model of pain. Second, models determine how health care professionals go about treating patients in pain, including choice of diagnostic procedures and treatment modalities as well as judgments regarding the efficacy of these procedures. Third, models determine how each individual (scientists, health care professionals, and lay people alike) appraises, responds to, and copes with his or her own experience of pain. Fourth, the ways in which people respond to pain in significant others (i.e., family members and friends) are determined by pain models. Fifth, models affect the manner in which larger social institutions and agencies (e.g., health care facilities, health insurance companies, and disability compensation systems) address the problem of pain. Finally, pain models constitute a starting point in our work with chronic-pain patients. Although treatment actually begins with the first assessment contact, we begin our work with patients who have been formally admitted to our program by discussing pain models. As stated by Turk et al. (1983), "Cognitive–behavioral interventions . . . begin by assessing the phenomenal world of patients in order to understand how they construe their presenting problems" (p. 181).

The development and elaboration of personal pain models are complex processes. Whenever pain is experienced, both sensory-informational and emotional schemata are simultaneously activated (Leventhal & Everhart, 1979). These schemata are derived from previous experiences with pain, become encoded in memory, and serve as a template to guide the entire process of pain perception including which features of the total situation are selectively attended to and elaborated. They also determine the nature of emotions accompanying pain and the behavioral expression of the total pain experience. Social factors (e.g., presence of significant others) also become an integral component of pain models. Particularly important are judgments regarding the cause of pain and what should be done about it.

Although, in one sense, every individual develops a unique model of pain based on his or her own particular set of experiences with it, we simplify matters and consider two general models that vary in specifics. The majority of pain patients and their families possess what could be called an "acute, peripheral disease model" of pain. This model is also predominant among most medical practitioners. Alternatively, we have chosen to advocate a multifaceted "biopsychosocial systems" model as being more appropriate for individuals with chronic-pain conditions as well as those with other chronic-health problems.

The remainder of this chapter is an attempt to make these contrasting pain models more explicit. In doing so, we believe it is useful to identify several contrasting dimensions that can characterize pain models. It is important to emphasize that we have no pretensions of convincing the reader of the "true or correct" pain model that should be applied to all patients pain. Rather, we believe that pain models and the approaches they generate should ultimately be judged on utilitarian grounds. This judgment involves the determination of how useful a given pain model is for a particular individual who is experiencing a particular type of pain or responding to another person in pain.

ACUTE- VERSUS CHRONIC-PAIN MODELS

At the most superficial level, the distinction between acute and chronic pain is usually based on the duration of a particular pain problem. Pain that persists beyond 6 months is generally regarded as chronic. More important than this simple, arbitrary temporal distinction are the underlying assumptions associated with acute- and chronic-pain models. Acute and chronic actually represent different conceptual models applied to illness in general. Acute-illness models tend to have four features according to Leventhal, Zimmerman, and Gutmann (1984): the illness is symptomatic and can be labeled (and different illnesses have different symptoms); the illness is caused by external disease agents; the illness is a short-term one; treatment can eliminate symptoms and cure the underlying disease process (p. 393).

A significant issue regarding pain is whether these same assumptions should be applied to chronic pain. This question can be restated as follows: Is chronic pain essentially the same as acute pain except that it persists over time? To clarify this issue we must consider how the acute-illness model applies to pain.

The Acute Pain Model

Acute pain is a temporary warning pain signaling physical injury or disease. Consider, for example, the occurrence of a toothache. Most people recognize that this type of pain is a signal or symptom of a pathological process involving the teeth or gums. As a result of this perception, the appropriate action is to visit a dentist. The dentist, who has been trained in an acute model of pain, responds to the patient's pain complaint as symptomatic of some form of dental disease. It is important to note that although the patient's pain served as a motivation to seek treatment, the pain itself is not the primary problem. Rather, the pain is a symptom of some underlying problem that can only be determined by using objective examination procedures (e.g., x rays and visual examination). Once the underlying problem has been identified, that is, a diagnosis has been made, appropriate treatment can be initiated. Appropriate treatment should eliminate the underlying pathological condition, and, as a result, the pain.

Acute pain is the most commonly experienced pain and the type of pain medical practitioners are best prepared to handle. Acute pain sensations are considered to be biologically appropriate, necessary, and usually accurate warning signals that directly indicate tissue damage or physiological dysfunction. Such pain is more technically referred to as nociception. Nociception refers to sensory input associated with the stimulation of specific nerve endings (A-delta and C fibers) that are triggered by tissue-damaging thermal, chemical, or mechanical stimuli (Loeser, 1982). The perception and interpretation of nociceptive input in the brain is what we ordinarily experience as pain. Although pain per se and nociception cannot be directly observed, the damaged tissue or physical dysfunction responsible for causing the pain should be observable or identifiable using objective medical diagnostic procedures. Finally, it is assumed that once natural healing takes place or appropriate medical treatment is completed, nociceptive input and pain should cease.

Chronic Pain

When pain persists or recurs over extended periods of time, at least two major aspects of the acute model are challenged. The first is the assumption that pain is temporary, and, second, that treatment eliminates symptoms and results in a cure. Nevertheless, many health care professionals, patients, and their families continue assuming some of the basic features of the acute model, primarily that pain is a direct symptom of some injury or specific disease processes. Unlike chronic-illness models that allow for multiple, interacting causal factors, acute models tend to assume single causes. Since pain is continuous or recurrent, it may be assumed, in accordance with an acute model, that it results from a specific injury that has failed to heal or from an identifiable chronic disease process. When medical practitioners are able to identify or at least label an ongoing disease mechanism, this basic feature of the acute model is upheld. In such cases, it is likely that there is no available medical technology to cure or eliminate the underlying problem. Although such pain can be considered chronic from a purely temporal perspective, some authorities, such as Crue (1983), refer to this type of pain as acute, since it functions in a similar manner to other types of acute pain. That is, nociceptive input from an underlying pathological process can be identified or is at least presumed to exist. Common examples of recurrent or ongoing acute pain include arthritic pain (rheumatoid or osteoarthritis), migraine headache, primary trigeminal neuralgia, and cancer pain.

Much more problematic are those cases in which pain persists without any clear indication of damaged tissue or disease processes. Medical practitioners who conceptualize chronic pain within an acute model are left with two alternative explanations. First, it is possible that the specific source of nociception is subtle or not easily identifiable. Consequently, some physicians resort to vague or speculative diagnoses. In other cases, the identification of the underlying disease may be considered beyond the expertise of a particular practitioner. Thus, it is common for chronic-pain patients to be referred to a succession of specialists if the cause of the pain is not readily apparent. Related to this is the possibility that pain is the result of some disease not yet discovered by medical science or of some pathophysiological mechanism not detectable with current technology.

The second alternative is to assume that the patient's report of continued pain is not based on any actual organic factors but is psychological in origin. In this case, the patient is presumed to be either consciously malingering or presenting a psychogenic pain disorder. From the perspective of the acute model, pain of psychological origin tends to be regarded as less real or legitimate than organically based pain. Popular terminology would suggest that psychological pain is in the head (i.e., imaginary) whereas physical (i.e., real) pain is in the body. Medical judgments regarding these two alternatives are usually based on inferences from the patient's behavior. It has been noted that health care practitioners have definite assumptions regarding how individuals ought to behave if their pain is truly organic (McCaffery, 1979). For example, if patients seem overly dramatic in expressing their pain, it may be assumed that they are exaggerating or trying to get sympathy from others. On the other hand, if the patient shows little or no signs of distress, it may be doubted that the patient really has pain. Judgments regarding the psychological origin of pain also tend to be made when it appears that the patient is using pain to derive some benefit (e.g., obtain drugs or avoid work). In short, judgments between these two alternatives are based on personal biases and assumptions rather than on any objective, scientific grounds.

For the individual who is actually experiencing pain, the second alternative is seldom acceptable. The vast majority of chronic-pain patients conceptualize their pain within an acute model. Since their pain has a perceived somatic locus, it is assumed that there must be an organic cause. The failure of medical specialists to identify the cause is then attributed to their lack of experience, competence, or expertise.

It is our contention that many types of chronic pain do not fit the assumption of the acute-pain model, which is predicated on a definite source of nociception. We also reject the dualistic assumptions implied in the concept of psychogenic pain. Psychological factors are involved in all pain, acute and chronic; however, they tend to play a much greater role when pain persists. We also believe that chronic pain is not the same as persistent acute pain. To clarify this issue, we will consider two other contrasting pain models.

PERIPHERAL VERSUS CENTRAL MODELS

The terms peripheral and central in this context refer to the two major divisions of the nervous system. Although it is universally agreed that both peripheral and central mechanisms are involved in the transmission and reception of pain sensations, at issue here is whether peripheral nociceptive input is necessarily involved in chronic pain. A related issue is the role played by the brain in the experience of pain.

Peripheral Models

The peripheral view corresponds most closely with the acute model of pain. Pain is essentially equated with peripheral nociceptive sensory input to the brain. Details regarding the anatomic structures, pain pathways, and physiological processes involved in the sensation of pain related to injury are well known to medical practitioners and are beyond the scope of this book.

In general, it can be said that the peripheral model tends to deemphasize the role played by the central nervous system. Traditionally, the spinal cord was thought to serve as a more or less direct, one-way transmission line from the peripheral site of injury to the brain. This became somewhat more complicated with the discovery of multiple ascending pathways to the brain. It is now recognized that there are at least two major ascending systems—the phylogenetically older paleo-spinothalamic, spinoreticular system and the newer neospinothalamic system. It is further recognized that multiple brain structures including the reticular formation, limbic system, thalamus, and cerebral cortex are all involved in the perception of pain. Nevertheless, traditional peripheral views tend to assign a relatively passive role to the spinal cord and brain. More simply put, the spinal cord conveys the message, and the brain receives the message. Lay people with little or no knowledge of the nervous system also tend to have a peripheral conception of pain. Although many are aware of the fact that ultimately it is the brain that receives pain messages, it is generally believed that the quality and intensity of the pain are determined solely at the site of injury or disease (i.e., at the periphery).

The idea that the brain passively receives nociceptive input from the periphery was significantly challenged by Melzack and Wall's (1965) "gate-control theory." Based on more recent discoveries in the neurophysiology of pain, they proposed a gatelike mechanism in the dorsal horns of the spinal cord that modulates the flow of neural impulses from the periphery to the brain. One significant component of their theory was a recognition that the brain itself can exert powerful influences on this gate system via descending efferent fibers. Consequently, "it is possible for brain activities subserving attention, emotion, and memories of prior experience to exert control over the sensory input" (Melzack & Wall, 1982, pp. 230-231).

Although some details of their original theory have been modified, the basic ideas of the gate-control theory are now generally accepted by the scientific community. Consequently, a much more significant role has been given to central nervous system factors in the experience of pain (both acute and chronic). The implications of this theory, however, are not generally known by the lay public and are often ignored by medical practitioners who have been trained in a peripheral model of pain.

Central Models

The central model of pain has been articulated by Crue (1983), who maintains that all chronic pain is primarily subserved by central mechanisms. In his classification scheme, he regards all forms of peripheral nociception as acute pain irrespective of temporal duration. Chronic pain is centrally generated pain produced by abnormalities within the mind/ brain system. These abnormalities may be caused by damage within the central nervous system itself (e.g., the thalamic pain syndrome following a stroke), unknown genetic factors, or they may result from psychological abnormalities operating in an otherwise normal brain. In many cases, the pain may have begun as a result of some peripheral injury; however, the persistence of pain after the injury has healed is likely the result of psychological factors. How this process occurs is poorly understood. It may involve interactions among factors in early psychological development, current environmental events, and cognitive labeling of physical sensations and other concomitants of emotional experiences.

Rather than making a sharp distinction between peripheral and central pain, we believe it is more accurate to recognize that central mechanisms are involved in all pain to varying degrees. The contributing role of peripheral factors lies on a continuum. With any given pain patient or pain episode, the question might be asked: To what extent is this person's experience of pain or pain behavior determined by peripheral nociception? Acute pain is more heavily determined by peripheral factors. However, even clear cases of injury can result in considerable variability in pain experience and behavior, depending on situational and cognitive appraisal factors. Chronic pain, in the sense of persistent or recurring pain, can also involve peripheral factors. For some these may play a significant role, whereas for others peripheral nociception may be entirely absent. In the latter case, it would appear that central mechanisms are exclusively responsible for generating pain experience and behavior.

The implications of central contributions to chronic pain are not easy for pain patients to accept. When pain is felt at a particular site in the body, it is very difficult to attribute pain to anything other than problems at that site. The only commonly recognized exception is phantom limb pain. Even though some people experience pain in an absent limb, they know that the source of their pain cannot be the limb itself.

The differential treatment implications of these two models are also considerable. For the peripheralist, the goal is to find and eliminate the source of chronic nociception. When the underlying source can be identified but not eliminated, the next alternative is to block peripheral nociceptive input from reaching the brain. This is presumed to be accomplished through chemical (e.g., neural blockade) or surgical means. If this cannot be accomplished effectively, the major remaining alternative is to dampen the brain's receptivity to pain through administration of narcotic analgesics.

To the centralist, the goal of diagnosing and treating the peripheral source of chronic pain is illusory. Since many types of chronic pain are not the result of peripheral nociception from a specific disease or injury, there is nothing to find, let alone treat, from a strictly medical perspective. Not only do conventional medical treatments often fail, but a consequence of their use is they exacerbate the very problem that they are intended to treat. According to Crue and Pinsky (1984),

> Patients should not be subjected to useless and repetitious nerve block, or irreversible orthopaedic and neurosurgical procedures that can lead to procedure dependency, increased dysphoria, neurological deficits, and increased suffering. Treatment should not include peripherally or centrally acting analgesic agents on a regular basis. (p. 863)

Thus, from our point of view it is essential to adopt a much broader perspective on the problem of chronic pain. One step in this direction can be made by contrasting the following two models.

DISEASE- VERSUS ILLNESS-BEHAVIOR MODELS

Following Leon Eisenberg (1977), we begin by making a distinction between disease and illness. Disease refers to specific disturbances in the structure or function of the body. The diagnosis and treatment of disease is essentially the function of clinical medicine. Illness, on the other hand, is a social–psychological construct. In the broadest sense, it refers to the subjective perception of not being well and the manner in which one reacts to this perception.

Disease Model of Pain

The disease model of pain is nearly synonymous with an acute, peripheral model of pain. Pain is a symptom of disease. Although it is possible to have a disease without pain, it is not possible to have pain without an underlying disease according to this model. In addition to being the model adopted by many medical practitioners, it is also the model assumed by most chronic-pain patients and their families.

Unfortunately for the disease model, the relationship between disease and chronic pain (a manifestation of illness) is quite variable. Many patients with chronic pain present no evidence of disease. The most common forms of headache (tension and migraine syndromes) are diagnosed by excluding the presence of disease. Specific indications of structural disorders involving the spine are absent in a large number of patients with chronic neck and low back pain. On the other hand, it is known that some individuals with spinal disk disease present no complaints of pain. In one large epidemiological study, 40% of those with no neck or back complaints showed radiological evidence of cervical disk degeneration, and 48% to 56% had evidence of lumbar disk degeneration (Valkenburg & Haanen, 1982). Clearly, there is a discontinuity between the presence of disease and complaints of chronic pain.

Illness Behavior Models of Pain

At least three illness behavior models of pain have been discussed in the literature. The first model is based on a sociological perspective and is concerned with role behaviors and expectations. A second model, described by Fordyce (1976), focuses primarily on overt, observable, learned pain behavior. A third model is considered cognitive–behavioral, since it includes the cognitive appraisal of pain sensations as well as the way in which one cognitively copes with pain.

The sociological perspective is based on Talcott Parsons' (1958) concept of the sick role. This refers to the socially expected rights and responsibilities of individuals when they are ill. The primary features of this role are as follows:

1. The ill person cannot be blamed for causing the illness. Thus, the person cannot be held responsible for being incapacitated in the first place.
2. As a result, the ill person is exempt from meeting normal role and task obligations.
3. At the same time, the ill person must view the illness as inherently undesirable. Consequently, there exists an obligation to try to "get well."
4. This obligation primarily involves seeking competent help (i.e., medical care) and cooperating with doctors in their attempt to help the person get well.

An important feature of this sick role is that it applies only to acute, time-limited conditions. Once people become well, they are expected to return to their normal activities and responsibilities. Conflicts tend to occur, however, when people who have a chronic condition adopt the sick role. Gildenberg and DeVaul (1985) suggest that the illness behavior of chronic-pain patients can be better understood in light of the acute sick role. For example, the repetitive and seemingly excessive search for medical treatment is part of the sick-role obligation to seek competent help. The willingness of patients to consume all kinds of drugs and submit to repetitive surgeries and other procedures is based on their perceived obligation to cooperate with medical management. The implicit assumption is that if "patients 'do their job', i.e., be willing and cooperative, doctors will 'do their job' and cure the pain" (Gildenberg & DeVaul, 1985, p. 18). Patients' desires to become well again usually refer to a complete return to the prepain status. Anything short of complete cure is rejected. Meanwhile, patients consider themselves excused from normal adult role responsibilities and entitled to receive care from significant others. The result is a regression to a more child-like state characterized by "marked increase in egocentricity, reduced scope of interest, preoccupation with bodily perceptions, notable increase in dependency, and oftentimes a demanding and manipulative insistence upon attention" (Gildenberg & DeVaul, 1985, p. 20).

A different perspective is offered by Fordyce (1976), who uses Skinnerian conditioning terminology to distinguish between respondent and operant pain behaviors. Respondent pain behavior is controlled by antecedent stimuli and occurs reflexively. As such, it is the basic paradigm for acute pain, since it refers to behavioral responses elicited by acute injury or disease. Examples of such behavior include vocal utterances (e.g., saying "ouch" or moaning), facial grimaces, walking with a limp, bracing reactions, postural changes, etc.

These same behaviors, however, can also become operants, which are defined as behavior controlled by consequent stimuli or reinforcement contingencies. In other words, operant behavior is learned behavior. Illness behavior and chronic-pain behavior are largely operant, since they are governed primarily by reinforcing consequences from the environment. Common chronic-pain behaviors include repetitive verbal complaints of pain, continual seeking of medical assistance, frequent use of medications, self-restriction of activity level, expressions of emotional distress, the filing of disability compensation claims, etc. In some cases, pain behavior is maintained by direct positive reinforcement such as attention and nurturance from others, receipt of disability compensation, the effects of pain medication, and rest from painful activity. In other cases, indirect but positive reinforcement occurs because the pain enables the individual to avoid aversive consequences. Significant reductions in many physical activities are considered to serve this function.

Although this model of learned illness behavior was an important contribution to our understanding of chronic pain and served as the basis for valuable new treatment approaches, we believe that a broader cognitive–behavioral perspective is needed. In fact, the very premise on which this chapter is based stems from such a model, namely, that the way in which pain is studied, treated, and reacted to depends on one's cognitive model of pain.

One example of a broader perspective on illness behavior was suggested by Mechanic (1962, 1978), and includes four interacting components: the perception of bodily symptoms; an interpretation of what these symptoms mean; the manner in which these symptoms are expressed; and what the individual does to cope with these symptoms. Symptom perception refers to one's attention to and perception of bodily sensations and changes that suggest the possibility of illness. Pain, of course, is a very salient sensation and likely to be noticed. However, the degree to which one is aware of it depends not only on the intensity of pain sensations but also on whether the person is involved in activities that distract attention away from the pain. Athletes, such as football players, may suffer painful injuries during the course of a game but pay little attention to the pain because of their intense involvement in the game.

In addition to perceiving pain sensations, people tend to make judgments regarding the cause and likely outcome of the particular symptom. The interpretation given to the symptom depends on several factors including the occurrence of specific environmental events, past experience with these sensations, and a variety of psychosocial and cultural factors. When the onset of pain is associated with a particular event (e.g., an accidental injury, dietary indiscretion, excessive alcohol consumption), it is likely that the cause of pain will be attributed to that event. In other situations, the onset of pain may be more spontaneous and not associated with a particular action or event. In such cases, the individual usually searches for more internal causes to explain the pain (i.e., some disease mechanism or physiological dysfunction). These subjective judgments also determine the emotional reactions to the situation. For example, the onset of abdominal pain can be attributed to a number of causes. Causal attributions of indigestion, food poisoning, duodenal ulcer, and cancer will likely evoke different emotional reactions.

Although symptom perception and interpretation are subjective, private experiences, symptom expression refers to the outward expression or communication of these sensations. Pain behavior includes, but is not limited to, the outward or public manifestation of one's subjective pain experience. Symptom expression includes both verbal and nonverbal behaviors.

The final feature of illness behavior is what the individual does to cope with the perception and appraisal of physical symptoms. One very important aspect of this concerns two additional models that will be discussed shortly, medical versus self-management. Essentially this involves the decision between seeking professional help or attempting self-treatment. From our perspective, this fourth component of illness behavior is of utmost importance, since it is a primary focus of intervention in our chronic-pain management program.

A related illness behavior model that has influenced our thinking has been offered by Leventhal and his colleagues (Leventhal, Meyer, & Nerenz, 1980; Leventhal & Nerenz, 1983). Whenever one experiences physical sensations or symptoms that suggest illness, there is a need to make sense out of what is occurring since such experiences represent a threat to one's well-being. As a result, people develop common sense representations of illness that reflect the influence of a small number of underlying implicit models or schemata. At least four basic components of such representations have been suggested:

1. Identity, which includes both concrete sensory features (e.g., "sharp pain in my abdomen") and abstract labels (e.g., "I'm getting an ulcer").
2. Assumptions regarding the cause (e.g., "I've been eating too many hot and spicy foods while under stress").
3. Consequences (e.g., "It will get worse if I don't change my diet and see a doctor").
4. Anticipated temporal course (e.g., "My pain will go away when the doctor gives me some medication").

In addition to the four cognitive components, these illness representations also evoke emotional responses. Depending on the interaction among these four components, people tend to develop one of three basic patterns of illness schemata:

1. An acute model with a specific cause and short time line.
2. A cyclic model that involves a recurrent cause and a longer time line.
3. A chronic model which involves multiple causes and the longest time line.

Of these, it appears that the acute model is especially preferable for many individuals even when they have a medically defined chronic disorder such as cancer or cardiovascular disease (Leventhal et al., 1984). As noted above, it is our impression that this acute-illness model is maintained by many individuals with chronic-pain conditions. One major implication of this tendency to adopt an acute-illness model for a condition that is actually chronic is that it often leads to maladaptive coping efforts.

REDUCTIONISTIC VERSUS SYSTEMS MODELS

Reductionistic Models

Acute, disease-oriented, peripheral models of pain are essentially reductionistic. The ideal of any acute disease model is to isolate a single basic cause and then devise a specific means to remove or repair that cause. The most notable attempts to approach this ideal have been found in the area of infectious disease. Specific diseases (e.g., tuberculosis) are caused by specific microorganisms (e.g., tubercle bacilli). Antibiotic treatment is effective when it neutralizes or eliminates the causal agent. The bulk of medical research is guided by a reductionistic model. Diseases ultimately can be understood and treated using the findings of biochemistry, genetics, and molecular biology. When this is accomplished, it will be irrelevant to consider how people behave and think in relation to any given disease. Although this reductionistic goal remains illusive for many major diseases, the goal is still being actively pursued. Consider cancer as one major disease category. Vast amounts of money are still being spent on attempts to find the definitive cure. This goal is very appealing, since, if reached, people will no longer have to concern themselves with restrictions on personal freedom through individual preventive health behaviors (e.g., refraining from smoking) or corporate actions that cut into profits (e.g., safe disposal of toxic wastes).

As applied to pain, the reductionistic view is seen in the way pain is defined, including the perceived causes of pain. Pain itself is reduced to a specific sensation as reflected in the following definition of pain offered by Wolff and Wolf (1958): "Pain is a specific sensory experience indicated through nerve structures which are separate from those which indicate other sensations such as touch, pressure, heat, and cold." This sensory experience could be further reduced to specific patterns of neural impulses (electrical–chemical changes) affecting isolated parts of the nervous system.

Reductionistic treatment goals for chronic pain commonly entail isolating specific structural defects presumed to cause these pain sensations and then correcting them surgically. This model is also highly appealing to most of our chronic-pain patients, since, if successful, they would no longer have to concern themselves with coping with pain since they would be pain-free. Unfortunately, the vast majority of chronic-pain conditions, including tension and migraine headache syndromes and low back pain, cannot be attributed to specific structural defects. As stated by Nachemson (1979):

> Having been engaged in research in this field for nearly 25 years and having been clinically engaged in back problems for nearly the same period of time and as a member and scientific advisor to several in-ternational back associations, I can only state that for the majority of our patients, the true cause of low back pain is unknown (p. 143).

Apart from curing or surgically correcting the underlying physical problem, another reductionistic goal is to find a means of completely blocking pain sensations while leaving all other systems intact and not producing any negative side effects. Thus, the perfect analgesic would be a drug that selectively blocks all unwanted chronic-pain sensations but has no effect on other sensations or physiological systems, has no tolerance effects, is not addicting, and has no adverse effects on cognition.

Systems Models

Rather than isolating specific cause-and-effect relationships between irreducible elements, systems models maintain that phenomena are to be understood by looking at relationships between or among interacting units (Miller, 1978; Schwartz, 1980; von Bertalanffy, 1968). Systems can be viewed as units or levels of analysis. Living systems can be looked at from multiple levels ranging from the cellular level to a far broader social systems level. It is also possible to arrange systems hierarchically. For example, a family can be regarded as a social system embedded in a larger social system (e.g., neighborhood, community). A family itself is com-prised of individual members. Each person within the family is also a complex psychobiological system comprised of various mental subsystems (Temoshok, 1983) and multiple organ systems, which, in turn, are made up of specialized cellular subsystems, etc. In other words, each system consists of interacting units linked together by some common property in such a way that the system as a whole is always greater than the sum of its individual parts (thus, a family is more than the sum of its individual members). According to Schwartz (1980), "the properties (or behavior) of a system as a whole emerge out of the interaction of the components comprising the system. Consequently, no one component 'equals' the whole system: All properties of complex systems have multiple causes rather than single causes" (p. 26).

Thus, a systems model would suggest that we will never understand pain by reducing it to neurophysiological and biochemical constructs. Pain and its expression are complex, multidimensional phenomena comprised of multiple interacting elements. Rather than being limited to specific sensory messages conducted by specific nerve pathways and triggered by tissue damage, pain includes various sensory-descriminative, motivational-affective, and cognitive-evaluative dimensions (Melzack & Casey, 1968; Melzack & Torgerson, 1971), as well as a range of behaviors aimed primarily at reducing the aversiveness of the total experience. Both the personal experience of pain and reactions to pain are influenced by familial and broader sociocultural systems factors. The experience of pain emerges from the reciprocal interactions among all of these dimensions. Additionally, the treatment of pain can be said to take place within a health care system that in itself is comprised of multiple interacting subsystems.

Although reductionistic analyses may be able to isolate specific biological triggers for acute pain, this approach is seldom able to account sufficiently for chronic pain. In other words, from a systems perspective, it does not matter whether a chronic-pain condition can be attributed to a specific cause and given a specific diagnosis (e.g., postherpetic neuralgia versus ideopathic low back pain). In order to understand more fully the origin of chronic pain and its effects on an individual as well as to devise effective treatment modalities, we must approach it from a multi-dimensional, systems perspective.

BIOMEDICAL VERSUS BIOPSYCHOSOCIAL MODELS

A distinction between biomedical and biopsychosocial models can be used to summarize and integrate the contrasting models presented thus far (see Table 2.1). The terms biomedical and biopsychosocial are drawn from a significant paper by Engel (1977). According to Engel,

> the dominant model of disease today is biomedical, with molecular biology its basic scientific discipline. It assumes disease to be fully accounted for by deviations from the norm of measurable biological (somatic) variables. It leaves no room within its framework for the social, psychological, and behavioral dimensions of illness. (p. 130)

He goes on to point out that the biomedical model embraces both reductionism and mind–body dualism. In its extreme form, this model has acquired the status of dogma resulting in the exclusion of all phenomena that cannot be reduced to physiochemical principles.

TABLE 2.1.   Contrasting Pain Models

Biomedical model	Biopsychosocial model
Most appropriate for *acute*-pain conditions	More useful for those with *chronic*-pain conditions
Emphasizes *peripheral* nociception	Recognizes the role that *central* mechanisms play in modulating peripheral nociception or generating the experience of pain in the absence of nociception
Focus on physical *disease* mechanisms	Recognizes the importance of *illness behavior* including cognitive and emotional responses to pain
Reductionistic approach to understanding and treating pain	Multidimensional *systems* approach to understanding and treating pain
Reliance on *medical management* approaches	Utilization of *self-management* approaches

As an alternative, Engel (1977) advocates a biopsychosocial model as a basis for an understanding of the determinants of disease as well as for the development of more effective treatment and health care approaches. Rather than focusing exclusively on biological determinants and somatic treatments, such a model includes psychological and social factors. Greater attention is given to the person with the disease than to altered biological processes.

Biomedical Model of Pain

When applied to the problem of pain, biomedical models are based on reductionistic, acute, peripheral disease concepts. Pain is a specific physical sensation that directly reflects physical injury or disease in the body. It is to be managed with physical assessment procedures and somatic treatment modalities. Basic research should focus primarily on delineating all the precise neurological and biochemical mechanisms involved in pain. Clinical research should be geared toward developing more sophisticated diagnostic tools to identifying exact pathophysiological mechanisms causing pain as well as discovering new pharmacological substances and surgical procedures to eradicate painful conditions. The setting for this research is the laboratory containing the most sophisticated tools of biomedical high technology.

Biopsychosocial Model of Pain

In contrast to the biomedical model, the biopsychosocial model is a broader systems perspective that includes not only biological factors but also cognitive, emotional, behavioral, and environmental factors. Rather than being secondary byproducts of more fundamental biological processes, psychosocial factors are inextricably involved in the phenomenon of pain. This multidimensional, interactional perspective is particularly useful in understanding chronic pain.

It is also recognized that a biomedical disease perspective may be sufficient to diagnose and treat many acute pain conditions. For example, an acute episode of abdominal pain may be diagnosed accurately as appendicitis and treated successfully through surgery. Even in this instance, we could examine the case using an illness behavior model to understand how the person initially appraised and reacted to the abdominal pain. However, it is understood that conventional biomedical diagnostic and treatment procedures were primarily responsible for successful resolution of the problem. Even though cognitive processes, emotional reactions, coping reactions, and environmental factors are always involved in pain, it is sufficient from a practical standpoint to view this type of pain primarily from a biomedical disease perspective.

It is with chronic-pain conditions that the biomedical model is often inadequate. Here it may be totally insufficient to restrict the focus to injured or diseased body structures. Instead, we must consider the persons who have the pain including their psychosocial history, illness behavior, coping resources, and the socioenvironmental contexts in which they live. In such cases, an honest and legitimate experience of somatic pain may be generated by central neuropsychological processes without any peripheral source of nociception.

MEDICAL VERSUS SELF-MANAGEMENT MODELS

Medical and self-management models represent two contrasting treatment perspectives. These alternatives do not necessarily refer to specific treatment techniques (e.g., medication versus relaxation training), nor do they refer to specific types of practitioners (e.g., physicians versus psychologists). Rather, these two approaches can be distinguished primarily with respect to responsibility for change and goals of change.

Under the medical model, responsibility resides primarily with a health care practitioner. Most often, but not necessarily, this practitioner is a physician. Within this perspective there is an implicit assumption shared by both practitioner and patient that the practitioner, by virtue of special training and expertise, will do something to or for the patient to alleviate the painful condition. The patient acts as a relatively passive recipient of these procedures, although it is expected that the patient will cooperate with the practitioner's instructions (e.g., take medication as prescribed).

The self-management approach places primary responsibility on the person with the chronic-pain condition. When health care practitioners are involved, their role is primarily that of teacher, guide, or resource person whose main purpose is to encourage or assist the patient in learning and making better use of pain self-management skills. Once instruction or guidance is completed, the responsibility for day-to-day pain management resides with the patient.

In addition to differences in responsibility, these two approaches differ in terms of goals or what can be expected. The most ambitious goal using the medical approach is correct diagnosis and treatment sufficient to produce a complete cure. From the patient's perspective, cure means total and lasting eradication of the pain experience. When it is acknowledged by the practitioner and patient that complete cure or lasting pain removal is not possible, the next treatment goal under the medical approach is reduction in pain intensity. It is hoped that, whatever technique the practitioner uses, the result will be significant relief from pain. Throughout this process, the patient's role is primarily to be a passive recipient of a particular treatment procedure.

Obviously, several other treatment goals may be held by the medical practitioner. These include various improvements in the patient's physical condition or psychological well-being. From the perspective of the patient, however, these other goals are usually subordinate to the primary goal of either complete removal or significant relief from the pain itself.

Expectations under the self-management alternative are generally more modest. Goals are no longer conceptualized in terms of cure. Self-management requires the patient to accept that cure is not likely, at least in the foreseeable future. It is further assumed that all reasonable medical diagnostic and treatment procedures have already been tried, and that complete and final correction of the underlying cause is not possible within the existing state of medical knowledge. The patient accepts the fact, albeit often reluctantly, that it is fruitless to continue searching for the right specialist (clinic or hospital) who possesses sufficient knowledge and skill to bring about a cure.

Reduction in experienced pain intensity may be a reasonable expectation under the self-management model. Unlike the medical model, responsibility for such relief resides with the patient. Reduction in pain intensity is then attributed to the patient's own coping efforts rather than to something done to or for the patient by a professional.

It is also important to note that self-management places less emphasis on attaining pain relief than is the case for the medical approach. At the time intense pain is experienced, the patient may focus less on attaining immediate pain relief and more on keeping calm to avoid exacerbating the pain through emotional distress. Furthermore, the patient who has mastered self-management may direct coping efforts toward surviving the intense pain episode rather than immediate pain reduction.

Finally, the self-management model involves a broader perspective regarding goals and expectations. Other aspects of the person's physical, psychological, and social condition are addressed and given greater importance. The patient and practitioner may work together in a collaborative manner to identify other goals and coping alternatives.

A most important issue facing the person with chronic pain is how to go about choosing between these two alternatives. Although there are no easy answers, we believe that both approaches are useful and relevant under different conditions. One important consideration is the particular stage in the course of a chronic-pain problem. Of course a person is not identified as having a chronic-pain condition until after a period of continued pain has elapsed (e.g., 6 months). Usually, one should not attempt to self-manage chronic pain until a thorough medical evaluation has been completed. It must be recognized that there are probably many individuals who suffer from chronic aches and pains without ever consulting a health care practitioner. Whether this is appropriate or not depends on the particular pain problem. Some individuals are probably better off managing the pain on their own. Others who attempt to self-manage their pain without consulting a physician are probably risking their health since the pain may be signaling a potentially serious condition that requires medical attention.

Our pain management program is concerned only with those who have already pursued a medical course of evaluation and treatment. In fact, we refuse to work with any chronic-pain patient until he or she has at least undergone a thorough but reasonable medical evaluation. Since we are in no position to determine what constitutes a thorough and reasonable medical evaluation, we work closely with physicians who share our basic philosophy regarding the limits of medicine and the merits of the self-management alternative.

The decision to switch from a medical approach to a self-management approach is often very difficult to make. Nevertheless, we believe self-management is preferable under two basic conditions. First, self-management should be used when it is clear that the medical approach, irrespective of the particular treatment technique used, is simply not working. Second, and more important, self-management should be used when continued pursuit of medical treatment appears to be perpetuating and exacerbating the pain problem. In other words, medical treatment is not only ineffective for many chronic-pain patients but also can have iatrogenic consequences that leave patients even more debilitated. These negative consequences can be seen in both physical and psychological areas of functioning. Unfortunately, many medical practitioners and their chronic-pain patients may not be fully aware that this is taking place. It is also the case that practitioners and patients alike may fail to recognize that self-management is a reasonable alternative. Of course, many pain patients have been given the following message by their physicians, "you'll just have to learn to live with your pain." Unfortunately, this often equates in the patient's mind with, "you're just going to have to grit your teeth and bear it as best as you can." It is our strong belief that self-management does not represent a grim alternative to failed medical treatment. Rather, self-management represents a positive alternative, an opportunity to regain self-respect, dignity, meaning, purpose, and joy in one's life in spite of having a chronic-pain condition. It means developing a sense of personal control over pain rather than being at its mercy.

Although the contrast between medical and self-management treatment models has been the primary focus of this section, we should mention an additional model that is discussed in the final chapter. We refer to this model as psychotherapeutic. It differs from both medical and self-management approaches in that the primary treatment goals concern problems other than pain. Although pain is the presenting complaint, it is considered to be symptomatic of other, more fundamental psychosocial problems that usually preexist the chronic-pain condition. It is further assumed that once these other problems have been successfully resolved, the pain will automatically diminish.

MEDICAL MANAGEMENT APPROACHES

Before turning to a more thorough discussion of self-management, which is covered in the next several chapters, we now review the major medical management approaches. In our experience, it is difficult to work with chronic-pain patients from a self-management perspective without first addressing their previous experiences and future alternatives regarding medical management. Because our patients have all had experience with this perspective, we can use this as a common basis for exploring their own expectations as well as their frustrations and disappointments with past medical treatment. Before we can even begin to promote the self-management perspective, we must make sure that our patients understand the legitimate uses and limitations of medicine.

Medical treatment approaches to chronic pain can be divided into two broad categories depending on the goal of treatment. These can be referred to as curative and symptom-focused approaches. The first category includes repetitive efforts to resolve, repair, or eliminate the underlying physical mechanism presumed to be responsible for the pain. This category of techniques fits within the acute, peripheral disease perspective. The second category consists of treatment approaches aimed at alleviating the pain symptom. Some of these approaches, such as medication, are aimed at temporarily alleviating the pain itself or other associated symptomatic consequences of chronic pain (e.g., depression, anxiety, sleep disturbances, muscle spasms). Others, primarily neurosurgical procedures, attempt to eradicate the pain permanently by destroying nerve mechanisms presumed to transmit pain impulses.

Following a brief discussion of the first category, we focus primarily on the second category of approaches, since these are much more common.

Repeated Efforts to Cure the Underlying Problem

The first category of approaches is always preferable since it would mean complete and final elimination of the pain. Unfortunately, the fact that the pain is chronic implies that this goal is often unrealistic. When chronic pain is attributed to some identifiable or diagnosable underlying disease process that is considered incurable, then no effort is made to eliminate the underlying pathology. For example, when an individual's joint pain is attributed to rheumatoid arthritis, no effort is made to cure the arthritis. Symptomatic management is considered the only alternative.

On the other hand, there are other cases in which an attempt is made to treat the underlying cause (following the acute pain model). Should the initial attempt prove unsuccessful, repeated efforts may be undertaken to resolve the underlying cause. Most commonly, such repeated efforts involve surgery. As discussed earlier, many people with chronic low back pain are subjected to multiple surgeries aimed at correcting the underlying spinal pathology presumed to be causing the pain.

Such cases of repeat failure are highly frustrating to both patient and physician. Each surgery is preceded by the hope that this will be the last one and that the pain problem will finally be resolved. Unfortunately, repeat failures often result in a widening of the gap between patient and physician, since there is a tendency for both patient and physician to attribute blame to the other. The patient, who is seeking medical solutions, has placed total responsibility on the physician. The physician has willingly assumed this responsibility but has not kept the implicit agreement to make the patient well again. Consequently, the patient may feel betrayed and blame the physician for being incompetent. Of course, the physician, who has applied his or her expertise and technical skill in a genuine attempt to treat the problem, may also feel betrayed by the patient. The physician may even have objective evidence that the surgical procedure worked as planned (e.g., pre- and postsurgery x rays indicate that surgery was successful). Yet the patient does not keep his or her end of the implicit agreement by reporting improvement in symptoms. Therefore, continued complaints of pain must mean that the patient's pain is psychogenic (i.e., not real).

This common scenario serves to widen the gulf between chronic-pain patient and treating physician. The patient, who sees no alternative, persists in an effort to obtain medical pain relief while a sense of frustration, anger, and resentment or feelings of hopelessness and helplessness continue to build. The physician is forced to devise his or her own strategies for coping with such unrewarding patients. Spending as little time as possible with the patient, referral to another specialist, and simply prescribing narcotic analgesics are common strategies. Fortunately, the growing popularity of chronic-pain management programs is becoming an increasingly attractive alternative.

Symptom-Focused Approaches: Temporary Measures

Most of the medical treatment approaches used with chronic-pain patients are aimed at providing relief from the pain symptom and other related symptoms. Although it is recognized that most of these approaches merely provide temporary relief and must be repeated, some of these do attempt to elicit permanent relief. The broadest category of temporary measures employed is pharmacological. Neurosurgical approaches, on the other hand, are typically aimed at providing permanent relief through destruction of nerves presumed to transmit pain. Such procedures are usually seen as a last resort after all else has failed. Besides medication, other temporary medical measures include nerve blocks, steroid injections, and various sensory stimulation procedures. A brief review of medical approaches used to manage chronic pain follows.

Medication

A variety of pharmacological agents are commonly used for individuals with chronic-pain conditions (Aronoff, Wagner, & Spangler, 1986). Analgesics constitute the largest category and can roughly be divided into two major categories, the narcotics and nonnarcotics. The narcotics act on the central nervous system, whereas the nonnarcotics do not. Whereas narcotics are very useful in the treatment of acute-pain conditions and chronic cancer pain, their use with chronic nonmalignant pain is controversial. It is our opinion that narcotics should not be used to manage chronic nonmalignant pain, since their negative consequences usually outweigh any positive benefits. In fact, as is discussed later, the typical p.r.n. ("as needed") use of narcotics for chronic pain can actually perpetuate and intensify the chronic-pain syndrome. The common prescription of these drugs produces some of the major iatrogenic consequences of the medical approach. Along with dependency, tolerance, and potential for abuse, chronic use often impairs concentration and memory, adversely affects mood and interpersonal relationships, leads to abuse of physical limitations, and generally undermines self-respect. In their discussion of narcotics and chronic pain, Gildenberg and DeVaul (1985) go so far as to state, "Of all of the things that are done in chronic pain clinics, probably the one which results in the greatest symptomatic improvement, when successfully concluded, is the withdrawal of pain medications" (p. 41).

Nonnarcotic analgesic agents are also used in the treatment of many chronic-pain conditions. Most of these, including aspirin, the major prototype, have three other major pharmacological properties besides analgesia. These are anti-inflammatory, anticoagulant, and fever-reducing properties. This group, commonly called nonsteroidal anti-inflammatory drugs (or NSAIDs), include both over-the-counter and prescription medications. Another nonnarcotic analgesic, acetaminophen (e.g., Tylenol®), has fever reduction properties but has no effect on inflammation or blood clotting. Because it has fewer negative side effects than aspirin, it is often the preferred analgesic for chronic-pain patients unless anti-inflammatory effects are desired.

Nonnarcotics differ from narcotics in that they operate at the site of the injury rather than in the central nervous system. The presumed mechanism for their action is inhibition of an enzyme that is responsible for the formation of prostaglandin. Prostaglandin is a chemical that sensitizes nociceptors on peripheral nerves to pain. Nonnarcotics also differ from the narcotics in that they have an upper limit in producing analgesia and thus are useful primarily for mild to moderate pain conditions. Fortunately, unlike the narcotics, they do not produce tolerance or dependence. Although these drugs are not as dangerous as the narcotics, there are acute toxic effects as well as negative effects associated with excessive chronic use. These include adverse effects on the gastrointestinal system (e.g., upper GI bleeding, erosive gastritis, and gastric ulceration) and renal system (e.g., nephritis and kidney failure).

Along with the analgesics, a number of other drugs are used with chronic-pain patients. Antianxiety agents, such as diazepam (Valium), may be used to reduce muscle tension, muscle spasms, and anxiety associated with chronic pain. These drugs share some of the negative features of the narcotics in that they can produce tolerance, dependency, and adverse effects on mental processes. Several other drugs that are chemically related to tranquilizers are labeled as central muscle relaxants even though they do not act directly on skeletal muscles. Since sleep disturbance often accompanies chronic-pain syndromes, sleep medications (hypnotics) are sometimes used. Most authorities recommend against the use of hypnotics and sedatives for chronic nonmalignant pain because of their potential for abuse and the fact that they may prolong sleep disturbance.

Antidepressant medications, especially the tricyclics, have become popular as adjuncts in managing chronic-pain conditions. Since depression and chronic pain so often coexist, their use is obvious. In addition to their antidepressant actions, they are thought to have analgesic effects through their effects on common biochemical substrates of pain and depression (Ward, 1986; Ward et al., 1982). Some also have sedative effects and can be useful in managing insomnia. Although antidepressants may be useful for some chronic-pain patients, they should be chosen carefully, and their effects should be monitored closely.

A variety of other chemical agents have been used with specific chronic-pain conditions such as migraine (e.g., ergot compounds, β blockers, serotonin inhibitors, and calcium-blocking agents). None of these drugs is completely effective with all patients, and many have several undesirable side effects.

One issue that should not be forgotten when evaluating any of these drugs is the role played by expectancy or placebo effect. Although this subject has been discussed by several others (Beecher, 1955; Evans, 1981; Shapiro & Morris, 1978; Spiro, 1986), we would point out that the placebo effect refers to more than obtaining pain relief following administration of an inactive substance (i.e., the so-called "sugar pill"). Rather, the usefulness of any treatment, pharmacological or otherwise, is influenced by patient expectations regarding the effectiveness of the given treatment. Clearly, within Western culture, there is a strong expectation that pain relief can be obtained through medication.

Although this positive expectation undoubtedly plays a role in the effectiveness of various pain medications, it is also responsible for some of the iatrogenic consequences of medical management. In addition to the many negative side effects already mentioned, it should be noted that medications reinforce patients' dependence on external agents for pain control. Their beneficial effects are almost always attributed solely to the specific chemical properties of the particular drug rather than to patient expectations. Consequently, patients learn to rely less on their own coping efforts and coping resources. As self-efficacy erodes and chronic pain continues, the patient sees no alternative but to seek more powerful chemicals or risky surgical procedures.

Physicians, for example, often feel pressured by their patients to prescribe more potent narcotics (e.g., "Doc, this pain is killing me, can't you give me something stronger?"). In order to alleviate the physician's concerns regarding addiction, the patient may add, "I really don't like having to take these narcotics, but I just have to take them because they are the only thing that helps." Many chronic-pain patients become physically and psychologically dependent on narcotics while concurrently denying their addiction. Since physicians vary considerably in their willingness to prescribe narcotics to those with chronic nonmalignant pain conditions, patients become skilled in finding those physicians with more liberal prescribing practices. According to a recent report by a national panel of experts convened by the National Institute of Health, there is a definite need for physicians to seek alternatives to narcotic analgesics when treating those with chronic nonmalignant pain problems.

Nerve Blocks

Another medical approach to chronic pain, used primarily by anesthesiologists, is the injection of drugs that supposedly block the ability of particular nerves to transmit pain impulses. Although considered a temporary measure, clinical experience has indicated that some patients experience pain relief well beyond the actual chemical blockade. Various chemical agents have been used. These include normal saline, anesthetic agents, corticosteroids, and chemicals that destroy nerves (neurolytic agents). The first three types are only briefly mentioned here, since neurolytics are more closely related to neurosurgical approaches (to be discussed later).

Local injections of anesthetics or steroids are used for certain pain conditions associated with inflammation (e.g., bursitis and tendinitis). So-called myofascial pain syndromes are often treated by trigger-point injections of a local anesthetic agent or saline. Another popular but controversial procedure is the epidural nerve block in which an anesthetic or steroid agent is injected into the epidural space surrounding the spinal cord. Finally, injection of anesthetic agents has been used to produce blockade in the sympathetic nervous system. These sympathetic blocks have been used for a group of pain syndromes often referred to as reflex sympathetic dystrophies (e.g., causalgias, thalamic syndrome, phantom limb pain, pain associated with spinal cord injury).

The value of these various nerve-block techniques in chronic pain continues to be debated. As noted above, some patients do derive significant benefit even beyond the pharmacological actions of the particular drug. The exact mechanisms for longer-term pain relief are not clearly understood. Many other patients fail to obtain relief beyond a few hours or days; thus, for them, the value of such efforts to treat chronic pain is very limited. In fact, this approach has become less popular in recent years (Brena & Hammonds, 1983). Irrespective of their value in providing pain relief, some have argued that these blocks have considerable diagnostic value. For example, it has been suggested that they can be used to distinguish organically based pain from pain arising from primarily psychological determinants (Morse, 1983). Occasionally, they are used as a prelude to destructive neurosurgical procedures. Here the assumption is made that if pain can be eliminated temporarily through injection of an anesthetic agent into a specific nerve, then total destruction of that nerve will permanently eradicate the pain. As we discuss shortly, this idea often proves illusory.

In addition to adverse physiological consequences, nerve blocks can reinforce patients' dependence on medical intervention, undermining beliefs in their own ability to manage chronic pain. Nevertheless, it has been asserted that many individuals with chronic pain are unable to accept the fact that their pain is the result of interacting variables including psychological factors (Brena & Hammonds, 1983). These patients, who rigidly cling to the medical model of pain, may be helped by nerve-block procedures, since they legitimize the medical nature of their problem (even when there is no clear evidence of nociception). Furthermore, these patients are able to attribute pain relief to a conventional medical procedure that fits more closely with their original expectations. Unfortunately, those individuals whose chronic pain is strongly associated with psychological variables may also be the very ones for whom nerve-block procedures are least effective.

Sensory Stimulation Techniques

Sensory stimulation refers to a miscellaneous group of techniques, ancient and modern, that relieve pain by producing some form of sensory input to the spinal cord and brain (Melzack & Wall, 1982). The most well-known ancient technique in this category is acupuncture. Others include cupping, scarification, and cauterization. Cupping refers to the use of a hot glass cup that is inverted and pressed over the painful area. As the air in the cup cools and contracts, the skin is sucked up into the resulting vacuum. Scarification involved cutting the skin with a sharp instrument, and cauterization involved burning the skin with a hot iron rod. Although these latter techniques are no longer used, there has been considerable interest in the use of acupuncture, a technique used in China for about 2,000 years. In spite of dramatic demonstrations of its use in surgery with carefully selected patients, its efficacy for most chronic-pain conditions has yet to be demonstrated. For example, Mendelson et al. (1983) found the technique to be no more effective than a placebo in a group of patients with chronic low back pain.

More modern examples of sensory stimulation techniques are those procedures commonly used by rehabilitation medicine physicians (physiatrists), physical therapists, and chiropractors. Various forms of massage and manual manipulations (e.g., stretching, twisting, and pulling) are used by a variety of practitioners for painful conditions. Spinal manipulation as performed by chiropractors is a particularly popular type of treatment sought by those with chronic back pain. Although the theory on which it is based is questionable, and the research evidence for its effectiveness is mixed (e.g., Crelin, 1973; Doran & Newell, 1975; Goldstine, 1975), there is no question that some people report temporary pain relief. It is interesting to note that one study found that patients were more happy or satisfied with the personal care received by chiropractors than patients receiving care by physicians (Kane, Olsen, Leymaster, Woolley, & Fisher, 1974).

Heat is another commonly used method of treating pain. Superficial heat can be applied through use of heating pads, various liniments, and mustard plasters. Other heating approaches include hot baths and showers, saunas, and use of hot tubs. Techniques used to produce local deep heat include ultrasound (employing high-frequency pressure waves) and diathermy (using electromagnetic radiation). Cold is another procedure used to relieve pain. Ice packs and ice massage can make an area feel numb or even produce an aching burning pain. Vapocoolant sprays are often used in combination with manual stretching of various limbs.

Finally, there has been considerable interest in various electrical stimulation techniques. Electrical stimulation can be applied superficially through transcutaneous electrical nerve stimulation (TENS). In this commonly used procedure, electrodes are attached to the surface of the skin, and a mild electric current is applied by a small, easily carried, battery-operated stimulator. Although TENS is quite effective for those with peripheral nerve injuries, it is much less effective for the majority of chronic-pain patients, especially those with concurrent psychosocial problems and no clearly identified peripheral source of nociception (Long, 1983).

Electrodes can also be implanted surgically, enabling one to stimulate parts of the central nervous system. One such procedure involves stimulation of the sensory nerve roots as they enter the spinal cord (dorsal column stimulators). Even more radical surgical implantation procedures involving direct stimulation of the brain have been attempted in cases of severe chronic pain. Although these surgical implantation procedures have resulted in at least temporary relief from pain, there is no clear evidence at this point that the benefits outweigh the risks.

Nevertheless, many of the other sensory stimulation techniques can be effective, and, even if they are not, there is little risk of harm. The exact mechanisms for their effectiveness are not clearly understood; however, Melzack and Wall (1982) suggest neurophysiological mechanisms shared in common by many of these techniques. This general mechanism, called hyperstimulation analgesia, is explained with reference to their gate-control theory of pain.

Finally, it should be noted that these sensory stimulation techniques vary with regard to their relationship to the medical model. Some techniques can only be obtained by consulting a health care professional (e.g., acupuncture, spinal manipulation, ultrasound), whereas others can easily be self-administered (e.g., heating pads, hot baths, ice packs) or obtained through the assistance of a family member (e.g., massage). Still another technique, TENS, can be easily self-administered but only after it is obtained through a physician's order. Obviously, our bias is in favor of safe procedures that can be self-administered. Such procedures have an advantage over the other medical procedures in that they can more easily enhance one's personal sense of control over chronic pain as opposed to reliance on a health care expert.

Neurosurgical Procedures

Some of the most extreme methods aimed at control of chronic pain have been developed by neurosurgeons. A variety of procedures have been used to destroy nerves or parts of the nervous system (neurolysis) with the goal of preventing the transmission or perception of pain (Melzack & Wall, 1982). These procedures have involved destruction of specific peripheral nerves, nerve roots close to their junction with the spinal cord (rhizotomy), nerve tracts within the spinal cord (cordotomy), parts of the sympathetic nervous system (sympathectomy), and parts of the brain itself using stereotaxic techniques and psychosurgery (e.g., frontal lobotomy and lobectomy). Such approaches have tended to be used only in extreme cases with patients who have failed to respond to other medical approaches such as medication.

The results of these approaches have not only been very disappointing but have sometimes led to "complications" whereby the patient ended up clinically worse than before surgery. Those patients who do obtain pain relief are often disappointed to find that the effects are temporary. Of course with some patients (e.g., those with terminal cancer), temporary procedures such as cordotomies may be justified. Unfortunately, for others the frequent occurrence of adverse consequences has made even temporary relief a risky venture. Loss of sensations other than pain and paralysis of various muscles have occurred. Some patients, through a process called "denervation hypersensitivity," have eventually developed worse pains as a result of nerve damage produced by the neurosurgical procedure (Melzack & Wall, 1982). Although research with these neurolytic approaches continues, many neurosurgeons are strongly opposed to their use with chronic nonmalignant-pain patients. Consequently, the use of these procedures has declined in recent years.

Psychological Approaches

We would like to conclude this section on medical treatment procedures by pointing out that psychological approaches can also be used within a medical management model. As stated earlier, our distinction between medical and self-management is not made in terms of specific techniques but rather the manner in which these techniques are used and cognitively appraised.

Two notable examples of psychological treatment approaches that have been used within a medical model are hypnosis and biofeedback. Both are generally viewed, by professionals and laypeople alike, as technical procedures applied to patients by professionals who have received special training in their use. In both cases, the patient may assume a relatively passive role as recipient of suggestions from a hypnotist or feedback from a complicated piece of equipment. It is commonly assumed that something is being done to the patient that will alleviate his or her pain. Biofeedback fits the medical model particularly well when it aims at directly altering physiological factors presumed to generate pain in the first place (Dolce & Raczynski, 1985; Turner & Chapman, 1982).

We believe that both procedures do have value in chronic-pain management. However, as is discussed in Chapter 7, we attempt to make use of them within a self-management framework. The key issue is how they are presented to the patient. We try to demystify the process of hypnosis and define it as something patients are already familiar with. We also define all hypnosis as "self-hypnosis," emphasizing that patients must be open and receptive in order for suggestions to work and that patients are in complete control at all times. Our stated goal is to teach patients some hypnotic strategies that they can eventually use on their own. Biofeedback training is also presented as a means whereby they can learn more about their own physiological responses and use this knowledge to gain greater control over their physical manifestations of tension. Connection to a machine is to be regarded as a temporary training tool, much like training wheels on a bicycle, that will be discarded when the patient can demonstrate control on his or her own.

Our primary concern is that whatever pain management technique patients use, the results will be attributed to their own efforts rather than to a procedure administered to them by a health care professional. From a cognitive point of view, we regard treatment success as increased self-efficacy in a patient's ability to manage pain rather than reductions in reported pain intensity. Some of our most successful patients report no change in average pain intensity while at the same time they claim a much greater sense of control not only over pain but over their lives in general. As is discussed in the chapter to follow, we consider the perception of control to be an essential component of treatment success.

SUMMARY

This chapter began with the premise that people develop conceptual models of pain enabling them to make sense out of their own pain experience as well as observed pain behavior in others. In addition to guiding people in their responses to pain, models determine the methods health care professionals use to diagnose and treat patients in pain. Although the word pain is used to describe any number of unpleasant experiences, our concern is with models of somatic pain. Most occurrences of somatic pain are time-limited and attributable to a specific injury or disease process. This type of pain fits the assumptions of an acute, peripheral disease model. Those with chronic pain, on the other hand, often fail to meet the assumptions of an acute disease model, resulting in frustration for both patients and health care providers. Chronic-pain patients are better understood with models emphasizing central (as opposed to peripheral) neurophysiological mechanisms and learned illness behavior (as opposed to disease) concepts.

As an alternative to a reductionistic biomedical model of pain, we advocate a biopsychosocial systems model that considers reciprocal interactions among biological, psychological, and socioenvironmental processes. Each of these interacting elements determines the way in which pain is experienced, expressed, and managed. This alternative model is particularly useful in devising treatments for those with chronic pain. Treatments arising from the biomedical disease model have generally attempted to eliminate the peripheral source of pain, block the transmission of pain to the brain, or directly dampen the brain's receptivity to pain. These treatments, including pharmacological and surgical approaches, neural blockade, neurolytic and stereotaxic methods, and various sensory stimulation and physical rehabilitation methods tend to fail, particularly with those who present a chronic benign pain syndrome. Since this syndrome is characterized by multiple psychosocial problems in addition to pain complaints, we recommend a self-management approach. This approach relies on a primarily educational model and places greater responsibility on the person with pain.

CHAPTER 3

Introduction to Self-Management Training

Self-management training, as discussed in this and the following chapters, represents a comprehensive treatment approach for those individuals who present many characteristics of the chronic-pain syndrome. These features include pain preoccupation, repetitive attempts to obtain medical relief, pursuit of disability compensation, attempts to convince others of their disabled status, narcotic dependency, depression, sleep disturbance, social withdrawal, interpersonal conflict, and general inactivity. In short, these are the chronic-pain patients who tend to get referred to specialty pain clinics. At the same time, it is recognized that not everyone who has a chronic-pain condition presents this syndrome. Many individuals are able to cope effectively with a painful chronic benign condition (e.g., rheumatoid arthritis) on their own with little expectations of health care professionals other than occasional assistance with symptom management. Others are able to derive considerable benefit from pain specialists who confine treatment to a specific procedure such as nerve blocks, trigger-point injections, physical therapy modalities, acupuncture, hypnosis, biofeedback, or relaxation training. These individuals tend to have relatively circumscribed pain conditions that do not pervade all aspects of their lives. They do not require a comprehensive self-management training program.

Actually, self-management training can vary considerably in scope. Biofeedback and instruction in relaxation techniques can be viewed as self-management training, since they involve teaching patients specific skills that they are expected to practice and utilize on their own. Cognitive–behavioral programs, such as the ones described by Turk et al. (1983) and Philips (1988), represent broader self-management approaches. These programs can be directed entirely by psychologists.

The self-management program described here combines psychological self-management approaches with physical reconditioning exercises, guided participation in diversionary activities, and narcotic medication reduction. A comprehensive self-management program can be adapted to individual patients. Our preference, however, is for group programs that are not only more cost effective but also make use of the therapeutic benefits inherent in groups (e.g., mutual support and encouragement among group members, peer feedback, and opportunity to work on interactional skills). Although such programs can be conducted on an inpatient or outpatient basis, our experience is primarily with inpatients. Inpatient programs have the advantage of allowing greater control over environmental factors (e.g., social reinforcement) including supervised withdrawal from narcotic analgesics. Removal of the patient from the home environment reduces the presence of distractions and obligations to perform normal role responsibilities. This allows patients to immerse themselves more fully in a total therapeutic environment. Disadvantages include dissimilarity to patients' home environment, increased presence of cues for illness behavior (e.g., hospital environment, presence of physicians and nurses), and greater cost. Our own inpatient program runs 5 days a week, enabling patients living in the local area to return to their homes during the weekend. We characterize weekends as opportunities to put into practice those skills learned in the hospital.

Ideal preparation of the patient for self-management training proceeds through several stages. In this chapter we consider three primary stages: the initial referral process, preliminary evaluative and preparatory measures prior to formal admission to a self-management training program, and introductory procedures after the patient has been admitted.

INITIAL REFERRAL PROCESS

Preparation of the patient for self-management training should begin with the physician. It is always unfortunate when we occasionally encounter chronic-pain patients who seek admission to our program in spite of, or even over, the objections of their primary physician. The following is an example:

A.B. was a 33-year-old married woman with a 12-year history of chronic low back and leg pain and four unsuccessful back operations. When a fifth operation was recommended, she refused and instead requested referral to a chronic-pain-management program. She had read about such programs in a popular magazine and was hopeful that they would be beneficial. The response of her surgeon was to criticize chronic-pain programs, especially those with a psychological emphasis. Eventually, she found a sympathetic physician who referred her to our program.

The report of this patient, and several others we have encountered, indicates that some physicians are either skeptical of or opposed outright to self-management programs. In each case, the patient had a clear organic basis for pain complaints but was having difficulty coping with the condition. Thus, we can only speculate that one basis for these physicians' opposition was a common misconception regarding which patients are appropriate to be referred to a psychologically based pain program. The essence of this misconception is that self-management, or a psychological approach, is of potential value only for those whose pain complaints lack an organic basis. Those who have clear medical findings must be treated with somatic methods. The basis of this misconception is a narrow, reductionistic disease model of pain. From our biopsychosocial perspective, the real issue is how well the person is coping with chronic pain.

Patient ability to cope with chronic pain can best be determined by a physician who has followed a particular patient over time. After going through the acute phase, multiple diagnostic procedures, and unsuccessful treatments, it must eventually be recognized that the patient has a chronic-pain condition. At this point, the basic focus must change. Physicians who understand the problem of chronic pain and recognize the limits of their own medical training find it easier to make this determination without having to blame the patient or themselves. Once this difficult decision has been reached, the next step is to communicate it to the patient in a compassionate, considerate, forthright manner. Messages to be avoided are implications (1) that the patient's pain is imaginary or psychogenic, (2) that the patient is at fault for failing to respond to previous treatment efforts, or (3) that the physician is about to abandon or give up on the patient. Although some patients may refuse to accept the physician's statement that the problem is chronic and no longer amenable to medical interventions aimed at cure, it is our impression that the majority respond in a positive manner. In fact, many appreciate the honest feedback and may even feel relief when told the truth.

In addition to communicating to the patient that the condition is chronic, the physician must also carefully assess the implications and consequences of chronic pain on the patient's life. This assessment should include an evaluation of patients' thoughts and feelings regarding their physical condition along with perceived options and coping alternatives. Inquiry should also be made into the family situation, perceived social supports, employment status, and daily activity patterns. Changes in the patient's life following onset of the pain problem should be noted. A considerable amount of significant information can also be obtained from the patient's spouse or other family members. Those who have developed many features of the chronic-pain syndrome, as described in Chapter 1, are usually appropriate candidates for referral to a specialized chronic-pain clinic. Some patients, on the other hand, are able to develop adaptive coping mechanisms on their own without any professional assistance. Such individuals are able to minimize the disabling effects of chronic pain, refrain from narcotic use, and lead active, full, productive lives while still living within their physical limitations. These individuals do not usually require referral to a self-management pain program.

Those patients who do need special pain-management training should be properly prepared by the referring physician. Preparation includes reasons for the referral and what the patient can realistically expect from a pain program. The primary reason for the referral is that currently there are no medical or surgical procedures that can totally eliminate the pain condition. If the patient is currently dependent on narcotics, the reasons for needing to be withdrawn from these drugs must be carefully explained. In addition to the often-noted negative side effects (e.g., tolerance, dependency, interference with mental functions, and physiological side effects), it should be emphasized that narcotics are meant to be used primarily for acute pain conditions. Now that it has become apparent that the patient's pain is chronic, it is necessary to find alternative methods for pain management.

Information already obtained from the patient regarding the disruptive effects of pain on his or her life can also be mentioned as an issue that needs to be addressed in a comprehensive pain program. Particular care should be given to preparing the patient for a pain program where psychological techniques are emphasized. The patient should also be led to understand that the involvement by psychologists in no way implies that he or she is "crazy" or that the pain is imagined. The basic message that should be conveyed is:

The Pain Clinic is designed for persons just like you who have chronic-pain conditions that cannot be eliminated through regular medical or surgical procedures. The purpose of the program is to teach you methods to reduce or better manage your pain so that you can lead a more normal and enjoyable life. You will be evaluated by chronic-pain specialists who are familiar with your type of problem and will be able to explain in greater detail the kinds of services that they provide.

In other words, referral to a pain clinic should be presented as a very appropriate and positive step rather than a sign of treatment failure. Statements that might lead to unrealistic expectations of complete cure should be avoided. It is more realistic to inform the patient that many others with similar pain problems have reported considerable benefit from such programs even though they continue to have pain.

Finally, it is important that the patient not feel abandoned by the primary care physician. Referral to a chronic-pain program should not be seen as an indication that the physician is trying to get rid of a patient. The patient should be assured that he can recontact his primary physician after receiving treatment from the pain program. Even though pain complaints have been a primary focus, it should also be kept in mind that chronic-pain patients can have medical problems that are unrelated to their pain condition. Some of these problems are serious enough to warrant continued physician monitoring.

PRELIMINARY EVALUATION PROCEDURES

Considerable differences can be found across pain clinics in the degree to which they emphasize initial assessment of each patient who has been referred. Some clinics spend relatively little time on assessment and immediately begin treating the patient with whatever specific modalities are being offered (e.g., nerve blocks, acupuncture, biofeedback, hypnosis). Other clinics conduct extremely comprehensive assessments involving a series of thorough evaluations by a number of specialists (e.g., neurologists, neurosurgeons, orthopedic surgeons, anesthesiologists, physiatrists, psychiatrists, clinical psychologists, vocational rehabilitation specialists, and physical therapists). Our own program is somewhere in the middle of these extremes. We believe that in the vast majority of cases extensive, and very expensive, medical work-ups are both unnecessary and contraindicated, since they reinforce patients' hopes that a medical solution will be found.

Medical Evaluation

Medical evaluation should consist of a thorough history and physical examination (Gildenberg & DeVaul, 1985). In addition to establishing baseline data regarding the chronic-pain condition, this evaluation should determine the following: (1) whether all reasonable diagnostic and treatment procedures have been tried in the past, (2) to what extent the patient is capable of participating in an active physical reconditioning program, and (3) the presence of concurrent medical problems unrelated to the pain condition.

Psychological Evaluation

Psychological evaluation should include a psychosocial history and a relatively brief battery of self-report psychological tests. The primary goals of this initial assessment process are threefold. First, it must be determined whether the person is an appropriate candidate for a self-management program. Second, an evaluation is made of psychosocial factors relevant to the patient's pain condition. Third, an attempt is made to further inform and educate the patient regarding the purpose and nature of self-management training.

Until recently, psychological assessment of the chronic-pain patient has not reflected changes in our understanding of the multidimensional nature of pain (Turk & Rudy, 1987). Traditional approaches have regarded pain either as having a physiological basis or as being the result of psychological factors. When medical findings have been absent or equivocal, general psychological inventories such as the Minnesota Multiphasic Personality Inventory (MMPI) have been used. Alternative assessment paradigms such as those developed from the operant model focus on behavioral manifestations of pain to the exclusion of affective and cognitive factors that determine the patient's perception of pain. We believe it is important to view pain as a complex, subjective phenomenon, uniquely experienced by the individual. Therefore, in order to understand this experience, we must assess patients' idiosyncratic appraisals of their situation, their unique experiences of pain, and their coping resources (Turk & Rudy, 1987).

As the above ideas would suggest, we consider it important to assess patients by focusing directly on factors related to the chronic-pain experience in addition to using more general psychological inventories such as the MMPI. Rather than using the MMPI to obtain specific information regarding patients' pain problems, the MMPI is used to identify psychopathology that might interfere with their ability to profit from self-management training. As a more direct pain assessment device, we have made use of the Multidimensional Pain Inventory (MPI), previously known as the West Haven–Yale Multidimensional Pain Inventory (WHYMPI) (Kearns, Turk, & Rudy, 1985; Turk & Rudy, 1987). This questionnaire consists of three parts. The first part contains five scales that assess perceptions of pain severity, how pain interferes with one's life, life control, affective distress, and social support. In the second part, patients indicate behavioral responses by significant others to displays of pain. Three scales in this section measure punishing responses, solicitous responses, and distracting responses. The final part is an activities checklist that is divided into four subscales (e.g., household chores, social activities) and a summary of general activity level. The MPI profile is also used to categorize the patient in one of three groupings: dysfunctional, interpersonally distressed, and minimizer/adaptive coper (Turk & Rudy, 1988). The MPI not only can be used to formulate a description of the pain patient across relevant psychosocial dimensions but can help in the comparison of individual patients to other pain patients and in assessing treatment outcome.

The MPI may be supplemented by other psychological inventories such as the Beck Depression Inventory (Beck, 1978). We have developed a questionnaire that assesses the individual's perceived ability to cope with pain using various medical, physical rehabilitation, and psychological modalities (see Table 3.1). Called the Pain Confidence Inventory (PCI), the questionnaire requires patients to rate their confidence in their ability to self-manage pain. Brief demographic and medical history questionnaires are also used. Of particular relevance is the necessity of assessing previous pain treatment history and perceived success of such interventions. This information can help explain the patient's attitude toward medical versus psychological intervention.

In addition to assessing the pain patient, we have also developed a short series of questionnaires to be completed by the spouse. Included in this series are questions assessing depression, marital satisfaction, perceived impact of the pain condition on the marriage, need for marital counseling, specific behavioral responses to displays of pain, and coping responses employed. Information obtained can be extremely valuable in understanding the patient's family milieu.

The clinical interview is also a very necessary part of the comprehensive assessment. Our interviews focus on attaining a thorough history of the patient's pain problem. Understanding the individual's attitude toward medical treatment and medical personnel is critical because the patient who is still seeking a medical solution to a pain problem is an unacceptable candidate for a self-management program. Rather than attempting to persuade such patients to abandon this pursuit, we often encourage them to explore medical evaluations and reasonable treatments that have been offered before considering a return to our clinic. A second critical factor discussed in the interview is the patient's willingness to be tapered off narcotic medication. Because a primary goal of self-management is the elimination of narcotic use, a patient's refusal to be gradually reduced from this medication would make him or her an unacceptable candidate for the program.

Another focus of the interview assessment should be a thorough examination of the patient's present pain-coping strategies. Patients who have developed ways of distracting themselves from their pain and who have found their pain intensity to vary in different situations are already making use of self-management techniques. These individuals usually respond well to the self-management philosophy and are typically interested in improving coping skills within the self-management program. Patients who notice no fluctuation in their pain levels or who report continuous pain at the very highest intensity level are typically resistant to

TABLE 3.1. Items on the Pain Confidence Inventory

---

1. I am confident that doing regular physical exercise on my own and keeping physically active can help me to manage my pain.
2. I am confident that I can manage my pain *without* taking any medications for my pain problem.
3. I am confident that I can manage my pain problem *without* receiving any further medical or surgical treatment.
4. I am confident that psychological (mental) pain control techniques can help me to better manage my pain.
5. I am confident that I can manage my pain *without* the help of doctors.
6. I am confident that keeping myself busy can help me to better manage my pain.
7. I *do not* need any narcotic pain medications (e.g., codeine) to manage my pain.
8. I am confident that I can hold a job in spite of my pain problem.
9. I am confident that I can accept myself and feel good about myself in spite of having a chronic-pain problem.
10. I *do not* believe that physical therapy modalities (e.g., ultrasound, traction, spray and stretch, whirlpool treatment) can help me to better manage my pain condition.
11. I am confident that I can better manage my pain by effectively handling psychological stress and negative emotions.
12. I am confident that I can be reasonably physically active in spite of my pain problem.
13. I am confident that I can manage *severe* pain episodes on my own by using self-hypnosis or a relaxation technique.
14. I am confident that I can manage *severe* pain episodes *without* taking any narcotic pain medications.
15. I am confident that I can manage *severe* pain episodes by diverting my attention away from the pain and onto something else.
16. I am confident that I can manage *severe* pain episodes *on my own* by using some form of physical stimulation (e.g., warm shower or bath, hot or cold packs, massage, electrical nerve stimulator).
17. I am confident that I can manage *severe* pain episodes *without* going to a doctor or emergency room for immediate help.
18. I am confident that I am able to *prevent* the occurrence of most *severe* pain episodes on my own.
19. As long as I avoid overdoing it physically, I can *prevent* the occurrence of most *severe* pain episodes.
20. I am confident that I can *prevent* the occurrence of most *severe* pain episodes by managing psychological stress and avoiding unnecessary emotional upsets.

---

nonmedical treatment. The assessment of family factors is an important part of the interview, and we encourage patients to bring their spouses with them as part of the evaluation process.

Psychiatric and substance abuse histories are also obtained in the assessment. We do not accept anyone who is in the midst of an acute psychiatric crisis. However, many of our prospective patients are severely depressed. We do accept such patients if they appear to be interested in our treatment approach and if this interest has a noticeable positive effect on their mood. Patients in need of more immediate psychiatric help are referred to an appropriate treatment setting with the understanding that they may be sent back to us for reevaluation at a later date.

One of the more difficult tasks in the initial psychological evaluation is to identify those individuals who present significant psychosocial problems that supersede the pain problem. Even though pain may be the primary presenting complaint, we sometimes encounter those who also appear to be experiencing considerable situational stress. Some individuals use somatic complaints as a means of seeking help for psychological problems. Others may present long-term patterns of marginal psychosocial adjustment and personality problems even though they have never sought or received mental health services. As is discussed in the final chapter, such individuals may not be appropriate candidates for self-management training that focuses primarily on coping with chronic pain. Rather, they are more in need of counseling or psychotherapeutic approaches that address these other problem areas.

Finally, it should be noted that the initial psychological evaluation can be of greatest value if it also includes an educational component. Without directly confronting the individual's belief system, we inform the prospective patient about the self-management model and how it differs from the traditional medical approach. Prior to our interview, the patient is given written material describing the program activities and their rationale. This written description prepares the patient for the types of questions we will be asking. Some patients come to the interview with a high degree of suspicion, distrust, and anger. They may not be pleased at being sent to a psychologist for what they consider to be a medical problem. This issue is related to how well they were prepared by the referral source as discussed above.

Because the pain experience is totally subjective, we do not question the patient's report. The patient must be made to understand both why he is being evaluated by a psychologist and that it is not because we believe his pain to be psychological as opposed to physical. Patients can be reassured by being told that no one affiliated with the pain clinic doubts that they are in as much pain as they say they are in. It is pointed out that it is normal for chronic pain to affect one emotionally and that pain (and everything else in one's life) may seem worse and more uncontrollable when a person is depressed. Thus, the evaluation interview allows for the opportunity both to assess the patient's pain experience and to educate the patient regarding a new way for him or her to think about his or her chronic-pain condition. Even when patients do not seem suitable for our program, they often leave the interview with new information and a strong sense of having been accepted on their own terms as opposed to having been viewed skeptically. Occasionally, the positive experience within the interview may lead the patient to return to our clinic at a later date (perhaps after further medical evaluation) expressing increased interest in the self-management program.

CONTRASTING MEDICAL AND SELF-MANAGEMENT

Once patients are admitted to the program, the most important initial goal is to assist them in redefining or reconceptualizing their problem. Most chronic-pain patients, often with the assistance of their physicians, have defined their problem in such a way that it has become unsolvable. Pain is the problem. Physical injury or disease is the cause. The only possible solution is to find the physical cause and fix it. The person with the pain problem is incapable of finding or fixing his own physical cause. Therefore, it is the responsibility of the medical profession to solve the problem. Since the medical professional has been unable to solve the problem, the patient is trapped in an unsolvable dilemma. Adopting a self-management perspective requires redefinition of the problem in such a way that solutions are possible.

The first session begins with the suggestion that whenever anyone experiences pain, he or she has two basic options that we label "medical management" and "self-management." We then proceed along the following lines:

Medical management refers to seeking advice or assistance from a health care professional, whereas self-management means taking care of the problem yourself or within your own home. Probably the majority of pain episodes are handled through self-management. For example, do you think I went to a doctor the last time I had a headache? No, of course not. I just took a couple of aspirin because I knew from my past experience that this would help make the headache go away. In other words, I used self-management. In fact, I would guess that many of the common aches and pains that you have experienced during your life including minor cuts, burns, bruises, scrapes, muscle aches, cramps, upset stomachs, and so forth have been handled through self-management.

The point we are making here is that using self-management for pain is something that everyone is familiar with, at least to some degree.

We then raise the question regarding how one decides whether or not to go to a doctor when a new pain is experienced. This leads to a discussion of the criteria people typically use for determining whether a given pain episode requires medical attention. Examples of such criteria include pain associated with an injury requiring medical attention, severe pain, pain that persists longer than expected, unfamiliar pain, and familiar pain that is known to indicate a disease requiring medical attention (e.g., toothache).

Patients are also asked to consider the physician's perspective when someone consults him with a complaint of pain. A toothache serves as a good example. It is emphasized that from the physician's or dentist's perspective the pain complaint is not the primary problem. For example we might ask:

What would you think of a dentist who responded to your pain by saying, "just show me where it hurts so I can inject it with a local anesthetic and when that wears off, here's this prescription for pain medication?" Obviously, that dentist is guilty of malpractice. The point is that dentists and doctors are trained to view pain as a symptom of some underlying injury or disease. The problem then is to identify the underlying problem (diagnosis) and then direct treatment to that problem.

We then proceed to give examples of the acute model of pain that are amenable to medical treatment. It is emphasized that acute pain serves a necessary warning function that signals an injury or disease process. In other words, it has important survival value. Patients can be asked to consider the implications of being unable to experience pain.

It is then pointed out that acute pain goes away after the injury has healed or the disease has run its course. Acute pain is by definition temporary pain. It may go away on its own, without any medical intervention, or following medical treatment aimed at treating the underlying cause. Finally, it is pointed out that doctors are primarily trained to diagnose and treat acute pain and that the pain almost everyone is most familiar with is acute pain.

We then confront patients with the reality of their chronic pain: If pain ordinarily goes away after the body heals or the disease has run its course, why is it that you continue to have pain? Why haven't the doctors been able to diagnosis and successfully treat whatever has been causing your pain? To clarify this dilemma, we discuss three general types of situations in which the usually successful acute model of pain is unsuccessful:

1. Pain is caused by a known chronic disease for which there is no known cure (e.g., arthritic condition).
2. The presumed cause of an acute pain problem was identified and treated; however, the treatment was unsuccessful (e.g., failed back surgery). In some cases there have been multiple failed efforts to "fix" the underlying problem.
3. The cause of the ongoing pain is unknown or poorly understood (e.g., pain that persists long after an injury has healed).

Occasionally, we also encounter patients who attribute the onset of their chronic pain to an invasive diagnostic or treatment procedure aimed at an unrelated problem (e.g., persistent chest pain following a lobectomy for lung cancer). The bottom line in each of these examples, whether or not the cause is identified, is that medicine has been unable to effect a cure. Consequently, the only alternative left is to direct treatment at the symptom, that is, the pain rather than at the underlying cause.

Patients are then asked to consider what methods doctors have at their disposal to treat the symptom of chronic pain. This leads to a fairly thorough discussion in lay terms of pharmacological approaches to pain management. Various types of medications are identified along with their intended uses, benefits, and drawbacks. Categories discussed include narcotic and nonnarcotic analgesics, muscle relaxants, minor tranquilizers, sleep medication, and antidepressants. Particular attention is given to discussion of narcotics, since most patients have had some experience with them, and their continued use constitutes a major obstacle to effective self-management. In addition to discussing the limitations of the pharmacological approach to chronic-pain management, we believe it is important that patients become better informed regarding the various drugs they have used or are currently taking. Some have serious misconceptions regarding the purpose and actions of specific medications. Other medical approaches aimed at the pain symptom are discussed as well, including nerve blocks and neurosurgical procedures.

We have found that this initial review of the medical approach to pain is an effective way to stimulate group discussion, since it is a topic with which group members have all had considerable experience. It also serves to highlight the disappointment and frustration that almost inevitably result from relying on these approaches. It can be pointed out that the patients would not be in the pain program if medical management had been successful. Patients are reminded of their frequent cycles of initial hope followed by disappointment each time they consulted a new specialist or began a new treatment regimen. Eventually, feelings of futility, helplessness, and hopelessness can emerge that only compound the problem.

Throughout this initial discussion the therapist or group leader is attempting to communicate empathy and understanding regarding patients' histories of frustration and disappointment with medical management. Those patients who were referred to a pain program because their physicians decided to discontinue prescribing narcotics often feel significant betrayal. Not only has their doctor failed to cure them, but he or she is now taking away the only thing that offers any relief. Although this discussion often elicits considerable anger toward physicians, care is taken to avoid reinforcing global condemnation of the medical profession. Medical management has failed not because doctors are uncaring, selfish, greedy, or incompetent but because current medical science with its focus on acute conditions is ill equipped to manage a complex, chronic problem such as chronic pain. Patients are reminded that physicians also experience considerable frustration and disappointment when attempting to treat chronic-pain patients.

Self-management is then presented as a major alternative to medical management. Although no promises can be made that anything will be done to eliminate patients' pain, it is emphasized that those who have successfully adopted self-management are much more confident in their ability to control and manage their pain. They also appear much happier and report feeling better about themselves in general. Rather than perceiving themselves as being at the mercy of their pain condition, patients can learn how to turn the tables by more effectively controlling their pain as well as reducing its destructive effects on their life. Although self-management may initially appear much more difficult than medical management, the long-term rewards of self-management are much greater. Thus, when first introducing self-management, the group leader is attempting the difficult goal of stimulating hope and positive expectancies without setting patients up for yet another failure.

INTRODUCING THE BIOPSYCHOSOCIAL SYSTEMS MODEL

The foundation for self-management is the biopsychosocial systems model of pain. We suggest that more effective control over chronic pain requires a thorough and accurate understanding of the nature of pain. Dualistic notions that consider pain as either entirely physical or psychological must be abandoned. All pain involves a combination of *bio*logical or physiological factors, *psycho*logical factors (mental, emotional, and behavioral), and *social*–environmental factors. Continuing with both lecture and group discussion format, the leader discusses each element of the biopsychoso-

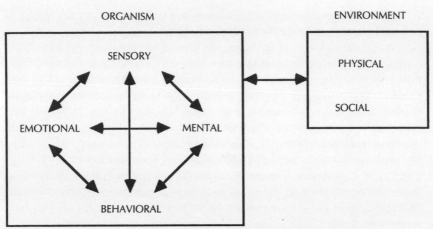

FIGURE 3.1.   The biopsychosocial model of chronic pain.

cial model. The diagram shown in Figure 3.1 is presented to illustrate the model. It is pointed out that elements are covered separately for the sake of discussion. In reality, each element interacts with and affects the others.

Physical Factors

To begin with, a distinction must be made between the experience of pain and indications of disease or injury as determined by a medical examination. Although pain can be experienced somatically (e.g., chest pain) or emotionally (e.g., heartache), the patients seen in chronic-pain management programs experience their pain primarily as a somatic event. They locate the pain somewhere in their bodies. A common misconception responsible for considerable confusion among pain patients and their families is the assumption that the experience of somatic pain must be accompanied by indications of injury or disease that can be clearly detected by physicians. Leventhal and Everhart (1979) refer to this as the "pain-injury" rule. Although injuries may result in pain, the presence of pain does not necessarily mean one is injured.

Patients are also reminded that pain sensations constitute a private experience. No one, including physicians, can directly see or measure another person's pain. The experience of pain may or may not be associated with observable indications of injury or disease. One can honestly report sensations of pain in the absence of any observable physical signs. Likewise, one can present clear, observable indications of injury or disease and yet report no pain. Private pain experience and public indications of physical damage may or may not correspond.

Related to the "pain-injury" rule is the "magnitude" rule that erroneously assumes that the greater the pain, the greater the degree of injury (Leventhal & Everhart, 1979). This common-sense idea is also responsible for much confusion and is especially a problem for those with chronic pain. With acute pain there tends to be a closer correspondence between the experience of pain and the degree of injury or disease, whereas in chronic pain, the relationship is much more variable. While clearly pointing out the incorrectness of the pain–injury and magnitude rules, it is important to reassure patients that their reports of pain sensations are accepted as valid, irrespective of medical test findings. Self-management is not concerned with locating, validating, or eliminating injury and disease. Rather, it is concerned with finding ways to alter the experience of pain sensations.

Pain sensations can be considered along several dimensions. First of all, they have a location. They are confined to some parts of the body and not others. Occasionally, we do encounter someone who reports "total body pain" until we ask how much pain is felt in the hair or fingernails. Second, these sensations have a qualitative dimension. Pain can be variously described as dull, aching, sharp, stabbing, penetrating, pressing, squeezing, burning, etc. Perhaps the most salient aspect of pain sensations is the intensity dimension. The most simple and direct way of describing pain intensity is along a single dimension. Patients may be asked to rate their pain intensity along a numerical continuum from 0 to 10 or from 0 to 100, with 0 representing no pain and the top number representing the worst pain imaginable. Pain-intensity thermometers can also be used. Another approach is to use verbal descriptors of intensity such as "mild, discomforting, distressing, horrible, and excruciating."

Pain sensations also vary on a temporal dimension. The specific location, quality, and intensity of pain sensations always fluctuate over time. Along with Turk, Meichenbaum, and Genest (1983), we attempt to help patients realize that pain sensations are not an invariant aspect of their existence. Sensations, especially their intensity, change over time. Self-management involves discovering those factors that seem to predict or influence the intensity of experienced pain sensations.

Finally, descriptions of pain sensations often include an affective dimension. Unpleasant, nagging, horrible, awful, and excruciating are words used to describe the emotional aspects of pain. Although the emotional component of the biopsychosocial model is discussed shortly, the point to be made here is that pain sensations are not neutral. Pain is an aversive experience not only because of the purely sensory aspects but also because it is usually an unpleasant emotional experience.

Mental Factors

We often begin our discussion of this component by reminding patients that an awake and aware mind is necessary to experience pain. A person who is sound asleep or unconscious does not experience pain irrespective of the amount of physical damage or disease. Although pain can have a negative effect on the quantity and quality of sleep, the fact remains that a person must be awake to actually experience pain.

In addition to basic awareness, we briefly review other mental or cognitive factors that are involved in the experience of pain, such as:

1. Focus of attention.
2. Memories of previous experiences with pain and events related to the chronic-pain condition.
3. Perceived coping alternatives.
4. Expectations regarding the implications of chronic pain for one's general well-being.
5. Attitudes and beliefs regarding oneself and others.

When first introducing the biopsychosocial model, we particularly emphasize the role of attention in pain perception. In Chapter 5 we discuss in greater detail how we present this concept to pain patients.

In addition to attention and awareness, another mental component is memory. Memory enables us to evaluate the meaning of pain. Whenever we feel pain, we automatically tend to compare it to our previous experiences with particular pain sensations. Because people maintain memory of their past experiences with pain, they are able to determine whether their current pain is a new, acute pain or whether it is part of the chronic pain. This is extremely important in responding appropriately to pain. An attempt to ignore pain through distraction can be a very useful or a dangerous strategy depending on whether the pain is chronic or an acute warning signal. In fact, the appropriate use of self-management requires the person to discriminate accurately between familiar chronic pain and sensations of new, acute pain that may require medical attention.

Along with enabling people to evaluate pain sensations, memory contributes to the meanings assigned to pain. In the process of growing up, inevitable experiences with pain can come to be associated with punishment, guilt, aggression, or receipt of attention and comfort from significant others. Memories can also contribute to many of the negative emotions that often accompany chronic pain. Memories of one's life before onset of a pain condition, circumstances surrounding a painful injury, disappointment with medical treatment, and adverse life changes associated with chronic pain all contribute to the ongoing experience of pain and suffering. At the same time these emotionally charged memories are subject to considerable distortion, filtering, and selective recall. For example, some patients recall their life prior to pain as having been very happy and conflict-free and life thereafter as filled with suffering and misery. Others selectively recall only disappointments and losses as though their entire life had been characterized by suffering.

Especially troublesome for some individuals are memories of a specific event that they believe "caused" the pain problem in the first place. These memory images may be vividly recalled at times of intense pain or emotional distress. Such memories often evoke intense anger when another person is blamed for apparently causing the injury. For example, some patients recall images of the physician who performed an invasive diagnostic or surgical procedure that initiated the pain. Others blame themselves for carelessness and failure to avoid a painful injury. The major point is that all of these selective, affect-laden memory images can contribute to the ongoing experience of pain.

Past experiences also influence expectations including perceived coping options. Some examples of varied expectations include the following self-statements:

"There is absolutely nothing I can do; I am totally helpless."
"If I can just find the right doctor (medication, operation, pain program, etc.), I'll be able to lick this problem."
"Even if the doctors can't do anything for me, I know I'll be able to live with this pain and make the best of it."

It is easy for most patients to see how each of these thoughts can have very different implications for how one feels. These alternative beliefs can differentially affect one's emotional reactions and overt actions (i.e., how one goes about coping with pain), and they can even influence the amount of pain experienced.

Patients are also reminded how chronic pain can have considerable negative repercussions on their self-worth, particularly when it is associated with physical limitations and perceived inability to be productive. In addition to attitudes toward oneself, chronic pain can also adversely affect attitudes toward other people. For example, some patients feel isolated because they believe no one can really understand their pain.

During the initial introduction to the biopsychosocial model, we make no attempt to cover all of the many cognitive factors that become involved with chronic pain. The role of cognitions including appraisal of environmental events and coping alternatives, cognitive distortions, cognitive coping techniques, pain-coping self-efficacy, and more global attitudes are discussed continuously throughout the program. In introducing the model the following general points are made:

1. Mental factors are *always* involved in pain perception.
2. Mental factors exert a tremendous effect on perceived pain intensity, the degree of suffering associated with pain, how one goes about coping with pain, as well as attitudes toward self, others, and one's future well-being.
3. By gaining more insight into the mental factors affecting one's pain, it is possible to learn more effective ways of controlling and managing the pain.

Emotions

Another basic component of pain concerns emotional reactions. It is emphasized that emotions are automatically elicited by pain and become part of the overall pain experience. The particular content of these emotions depends partly on the meaning given to the pain in terms of its implications for one's well-being.

Onset of acute pain is typically accompanied by general emotional distress that can serve an extremely important and necessary function. Acute pain serves to motivate people to respond to their pain with behavior that will promote or allow healing (e.g., rest, inactivity, seeking medical attention). Acute pain should not be ignored. Emotional arousal is an activating and energizing force that impels one to act.

Anxiety often occurs when the evaluation of acute pain includes a great deal of uncertainty. The person knows that something is wrong but has no idea what it might be. Fear may occur if the person suspects that pain is the result of some serious, life-threatening disease such as cancer or a heart condition. Fear also tends to accompany suspected diseases that may require uncomfortable medical or surgical intervention such as an acute appendicitis or a kidney infection. Anxiety and fear associated with acute pain often, but not necessarily, motivate a person to seek medical attention. Occasionally, the opposite phenomenon occurs in that the person avoids medical attention out of fear of what might be discovered.

Anxiety and fear can also be associated with chronic pain. Although pain sensations have become more familiar, and medical attention has been already received, some patients worry about how they will be able to handle pain if their condition continues to deteriorate. Fear of increased pain also becomes associated with specific activities leading to increased avoidance of such activities. Such fear and avoidance patterns can generalize to a wide variety of activities resulting in increased physical degeneration, depression, and pain preoccupation. Others experience fear and anxiety not because of the pain itself but because of what it may mean in terms of their lives. For example, anxiety may be associated with questions such as: "Will I ever be able to work again? How am I going to survive financially? What will I do if my condition keeps getting worse?"

One of the most common emotional states that coexists with chronic pain is depression. In addition to depressed mood, social withdrawal, isolation, low energy, apathy, and suicidal thoughts are common. Chronic pain can easily be viewed as an uncontrollable, aversive situation from which there is no escape. If the patient has adopted an acute medical model, pain is considered to be the direct result of some underlying disease process or the residual effects of an injury over which the person has no direct control. The only recourse is to entrust oneself to medical treatment. After years of repeated efforts to attain relief through biomedical treatment fail, the person learns to feel more and more helpless. Along with these feelings of helplessness, a sense of hopelessness can also develop. Not only is there nothing that can be done at the present time, it is unlikely that anything can ever be done to relieve the chronic pain and misery. Of course, helplessness and hopelessness are natural preludes to suicidal thoughts or efforts to escape through excessive alcohol use or abuse of narcotic analgesics. Depression has become a dominant feature of these patients' lives. Depression often becomes part of a vicious cycle that further intensifies pain preoccupation and maladaptive efforts to cope with it. In fact, a major component of the self-management of chronic pain is learning how to understand and better cope with depression.

Along with depression, feelings of frustration, irritability, impatience, hostility, bitterness, and outbursts of anger are common features of chronic pain. Chronic-pain patients are often perceived by health care professionals as hostile, angry, and demanding individuals. Disturbed family relationships, conflicts with health care practitioners, and ongoing battles with the disability compensation system are also common.

Some patients tend to project considerable blame onto others for their plight. Doctors may be seen as incompetent quacks who are only interested in making money. The disability system is viewed as grossly unfair and out to deprive them of their legitimate claims for compensation. Employers are considered to be totally unwilling to even consider hiring a person with chronic pain and disability. One of our patients summarized his feelings by saying, "People are stupid and don't give a damn, so to hell with them."

Others feel continually frustrated over their own inability to engage in many activities that they used to do. For example, as a result of chronic low back pain, the person may feel considerable frustration over an inability to work or engage in leisure pursuits that were previously enjoyed. Along with frustration, the person may feel generally irritable and bitter because previous sources of pride, satisfaction, and enjoyment are no longer considered available.

When we initially present the emotional component of the biopsychosocial model, we make an effort to point out the normality of these negative affective states when someone suffers from a chronic-pain condition. Rather than present them as signs of psychiatric disturbance, we emphasize that feelings of depression, anger, and anxiety are expected and common features of chronic pain. Patients are encouraged to give examples from their own lives that illustrate these common emotional reactions. This works most effectively in a group setting, since when one patient begins to disclose feelings of depression, anxiety, frustration, and anger, it serves to disinhibit others into sharing their own feelings.

In addition to emotional states associated with the experience of pain or adverse consequences of pain, patients are reminded that emotional reactions to other upsetting events or situational difficulties can interact with pain. In other words, emotional reactions to situations that have nothing to do with pain can nonetheless contribute to the pain experience. It is also important to keep reminding patients of the interactive nature between negative emotional states and pain perception. The reciprocal interaction between these two processes often creates a vicious cycle in which both are intensified.

When first introducing patients to the biopsychosocial model of pain, we treat emotions as a specific component of the model. As the program progresses and specific emotions are discussed in greater depth, it is pointed out that emotions themselves can be considered from a biopsychosocial framework. That is, in addition to the affective feeling state, emotions include physiological and sensory factors, cognitions, and overt behaviors. Social and environmental factors must also be considered. Environmental factors can trigger emotions, and the overt expression of various emotional states can have an impact on the person's immediate social environment.

Actions

This component refers to immediate expressions of pain, the various ways in which pain is communicated, actions taken to cope with pain, and changes in behavior as a result of chronic pain. We begin by making a clear distinction between the private experience of pain and public (i.e., observable) expressions of pain behavior. The failure to distinguish these two concepts can lead to much confusion for patients and their families. It is emphasized that the two do not necessarily go together. One person may experience considerable pain while showing relatively little pain behavior, whereas another may show a great deal of pain behavior in spite of little or no pain. Some overt expressions of pain appear to be relatively automatic, reflex-like actions. Examples include vocal utterances (e.g., saying "ouch" or moaning), facial grimaces, walking with a limp, bracing, stiff and guarded movements, rubbing affected body parts, etc. Although they may appear to be automatic and involuntary, we know that they can be influenced by social and psychological factors. Expression of pain may reflect family influences and cultural differences or, in some cases, may involve an attempt to have an effect on others. For example, occasionally our patients will limp noticeably when they know they are being observed but walk normally when they think they are not being observed.

In addition to these more or less immediate expressions of pain, patients are asked to consider those actions commonly taken to cope with their pain. These are also considered chronic-pain behaviors. Examples include seeking medical assistance, taking medications, restricting activity level, communicating to others that one is in pain, withdrawing from others, etc. In addition to these behaviors characteristic of the chronic-pain syndrome, many report attempts to engage in some activity that diverts their attention from pain. Pain-coping actions can be positive or negative depending on their immediate and long-term consequences.

Environmental Influences

To complete the biopsychosocial model, environmental factors are discussed. We begin by arbitrarily distinguishing between the physical and social environment. A number of features of the physical environment can interact with the sensations, cognitions, emotions, and behaviors associated with chronic pain. Living conditions, material resources, and even weather changes can influence pain awareness and how one goes about coping with pain. The social environment includes family, friends, coworkers, health care professionals, and an assortment of strangers with whom the person may come in contact. Other aspects of the environment include health care systems, disability compensation systems, and a whole host of sociocultural factors.

Environmental factors can differentially affect the various pain components discussed thus far. Some aspects of the physical environment appear to influence pain sensations directly. For example, many patients with arthritic pain report increased discomfort during cold, damp weather conditions. Those with low back pain may be affected by the type of mattress on which they sleep or the degree of lumbar support provided by chairs on which they sit. More important is the presence or absence of various environmental cues that can differentially influence attentional processes and pain perception. This subject is discussed more fully in Chapter 5.

Particular attention is given to the role of the social environment on cognitions, emotions, and behavior associated with pain. Pain can be influenced not only by the immediate social environment but also by the social environment in which the person was raised. For example, we may refer to some of the findings of medical sociologists such as Zborowski

(1952) and Zola (1966), who pointed out how one's sociocultural environment affects the manner in which pain is perceived and expressed. Of course, sociocultural influences are transmitted primarily via family rearing patterns. Children learn from their parents ways of perceiving and responding to physical symptoms and illness in general. Such learning takes place automatically, without conscious plan or intent, through parental example (modeling) and reinforcement.

Examples of how the patient's current social environment interacts with pain are also discussed. Particular emphasis is put on family factors. Patients are asked to consider how the behavior of various family members affects their overall pain condition. Additionally, they are asked to consider how their pain condition has affected their family life. For example, a patient may report increased irritability when his or her young child is playing and making noise. As a result, the patient may angrily punish the child. This is often followed by feelings of guilt for being so nasty to the child for engaging in normal child-like behavior. Other family factors such as marital conflict, role changes, and withdrawal from family activities are often reported.

During the initial discussion of this model, emphasis is usually placed on the negative interactive effects between chronic pain and the social environment. Although we know that the social environment can also positively reinforce pain behavior, this point is not stressed at first since it tends to evoke patient resistance. When the issue of "pain payoffs" is introduced, it is emphasized that this does not necessarily imply that the patient is consciously and deliberately fabricating pain complaints in order to elicit various environmental rewards such as attention, sympathy, and control over others.

Finally, the effects of deficits in the patient's social environment should be considered. Some of our pain patients live in near-total social isolation. These patients may be divorced or widowed, childless, or alienated from their children and lacking in any meaningful social ties. Some have deliberately isolated themselves, whereas others have become inadvertently isolated because their pain behavior has driven others away. Failure to initiate social contacts, repeated refusals to participate in invited social activities, or excessive pain complaints in the presence of friends can eventually lead to considerable social isolation. The implications of this pattern on the emotional, cognitive, and behavioral aspects of the pain experience should be discussed.

Additional Considerations

Other useful guidelines regarding the initial orientation and reconceptualization process are found in Philips (1988) and Turk et al.

(1983). Throughout this process, the interactive components of this model are repeatedly pointed out, especially with regard to the many vicious cycles that tend to develop over time. Most patients will readily agree that chronic pain has had adverse effects on many aspects of their lives. Consequently, the model is presented in a way that highlights the disruptive, negative consequences of chronic pain. As mentioned above, we initially avoid references to the positive consequences of pain (unless they are brought up by the patients) even though we know they certainly may be relevant. Most chronic-pain patients become quite defensive if it is suggested that their pain behavior is being maintained by positive reinforcement or that they have an unconscious need to suffer. The functional aspects of chronic pain are gradually introduced later in the program.

The overall goal at the beginning is to develop a good collaborative, working relationship, while helping patients reconceptualize their problems to fit the broad, integrative themes of this model. It is through this reconceptualization process that they can begin to see how change is possible. After reviewing all of the major components of the biopsychosocial model, we may ask patients to consider how much direct control they have over each component. Most recognize that they have little direct control over the sensory components of pain. More controversial is our assertion that we have little direct control over our emotional states, even though we may have control over the way emotions are expressed.

Mood states including depression, irritability, and feelings of anxious apprehension cannot be turned off or on at will. For example, if we are feeling depressed and someone comes along and says, "stop being depressed," we are powerless to directly change our mood state even if we really want to. We suggest that people have greater potential control over mental factors. However, there are significant limitations here as well. With regard to this domain, it is suggested that one can *learn* to exert greater control by practicing various "mental techniques" such as attention diversion, autogenic and mental imagery exercises, positive self-talk, and even self-hypnosis. Furthermore, one can eventually learn to exert greater control by closely examining automatic thoughts associated with various attitudes, beliefs, expectations, and the way in which environmental demands are appraised. This process is discussed more fully in Chapter 7. By far the greatest degree of direct control is over the action component. With the exception of a small number of automatic reflexes, we have the potential of voluntarily controlling virtually all of our overt behavior.

This issue of control can be summarized by pointing out that self-management training primarily focuses on changing thoughts (cognitions) and actions (behavior). Consequently, we sometimes refer to our approach as "cognitive–behavioral." This is not to suggest that sensory and emotional factors are any less important in pain. Rather, it is because of the interactive nature of the biopsychosocial perspective that change over these other factors is possible. Pain sensations and negative emotions are controlled *indirectly* by changing thoughts and actions.

Finally, when presenting this broad, integrative biopsychosocial model to patients it is important to keep the following points in mind:

1. Use simple, common lay terms and avoid professional jargon (e.g.,"thoughts" rather than "cognitions" or "emotions and feelings" rather than "affect").
2. Ilustrate points with examples drawn from common experiences of chronic-pain patients.
3. Encourage attention and active participation by asking the group simple questions (e.g., "What are some of the common emotional reactions that go along with having chronic pain?").
4. Encourage questions from group participants.
5. Avoid getting sidetracked on tangential or irrelevant issues.
6. Supplement lecture information with written materials (see Tables 3.2 through 3.5).

Rather than presenting a dull, abstract theory, we make considerable effort to make our presentation lively, practical, and relevant. Group discussion is encouraged while the leader tries to keep to the main points. A skilled group leader will attempt to modulate his or her presentation according to the atmosphere or mood of the group as a whole as well as the behavior of individual participants. For example, an effort is made to draw out quiet and withdrawn participants while gently restraining those who monopolize discussion or digress from the topic.

Presenting a Neurophysiological Basis for the Biopsychosocial Model

At some point in either the orientation process or later in the program, it is useful to present a simple neurophysiological model of pain. For some, this serves to increase the credibility of the biopsychosocial model. The following three interrelated aspects can be covered:

1. Multiple areas of brain function that play a role in pain perception.
2. The gate-control theory and factors that influence the gate.
3. The role of endorphins in pain perception.

TABLE 3.2. Introductory Concepts: Medical versus Self-Management of Chronic Pain

Medical management	Responsibility placed on health care professional
	Emphasis on physical procedures (e.g., drugs, surgery, nerve blocks)
	Greater risk of negative side effects
	Most effective with *acute* injuries and diseases
Self-management	Responsibility placed on the person with the chronic-pain problem
	Less emphasis on physical procedures
	Emphasis on emotional, mental, behavioral, and social factors
	Primary goal is to cope more effectively with pain and associated problems
	Very useful for *chronic* pain and other chronic-physical conditions

With a simple diagram of the brain, it is pointed out that different areas of the brain are automatically involved in pain. Arriving pain signals are relayed by the thalamus to the sensory cortex, which is able to discriminate the sensory components of pain. Concurrently, pain signals activate the limbic system, which underlies the emotional component of pain. Brain structures involved in memory are also activated. Pain is mentally evaluated, and decisions are made regarding what to do about it in the frontal cortex. Pain behaviors are initiated by activating the motor cortex. Each of these brain areas, which underlie the sensory, emotional, mental, and action components of the biopsychosocial model, connects with and influences the others.

TABLE 3.3. Acute versus Chronic Pain

Acute pain	Serves a useful warning function: symptom of underlying disease or injury
	Ends after the injury heals or the disease runs its course
Chronic pain	Pain that persists longer than 6 months
	May be symptomatic of an underlying chronic disease or may exist in the absence of an underlying disease
	Persists long after the initial injury has healed
	No longer serves as a useful warning function

TABLE 3.4.   Experience of Pain versus Pain Behavior versus Medical
Indications of Disease or Injury

Pain experience	Personal, subjective experience of pain known only to the person with pain
	Cannot be objectively measured, confirmed, or disconfirmed
	May or may not be accompanied by physical injury or disease
Pain behavior	Outward, observable indications of pain
	Includes verbal complaints of pain as well as nonverbal indications of pain (e.g., grimacing, moaning, limping, rubbing one's body, bracing) and pain-coping behaviors (e.g., taking medication, lying in bed, withdrawing in silence)
	May or may not be accompanied by the experience of pain
Medical indications of disease or injury	Confirmation of disease or injury based on physical examination and medical test procedures (e.g., lab tests, x ray, CAT scan, MRI, EMG/NCV)
	May or may not be associated with pain experience
Conclusion	Although there may be a clear overlap between the experience of pain, pain behavior, and medical indications of disease or injury, they do not necessarily go together. In other words, they are *not* the same thing. Failure to understand this has resulted in much confusion on the part of doctors, pain patients, and their families.

In addition to the involvement of multiple brain areas, it is emphasized that pain signals that have originated in areas of injury or disease do not travel directly and automatically to the brain. Rather, there exists within the spinal cord a gate mechanism which determines the degree to which pain signals are transmitted to the brain. When the gate is wide open, more pain signals get through than when it is closed. Generally, rather than being fully open or completely shut, it is open to varying degrees. The degree to which the gate is open is determined by two sets of influences. First is the pattern of sensory signals that travel to the spinal gate. Second, and more important for our purposes, are inhibitory messages from the brain itself. In other words, psychological factors that involve brain processes can close the gate to varying degrees.

TABLE 3.5. Biopsychosocial Model of Pain

BASIC CONCEPT:

A complete understanding of pain must take into account *bio*logical (physical), *psycho*logical (emotional, mental, behavioral), and *social* (response of other people) factors. It is impossible to understand pain using physical concepts alone.

CHRONIC PAIN:

Although psychological and social factors are involved in *all* pain, they are likely to become even more important when pain persists over time and becomes chronic.

ELEMENTS:

Sensory

This refers to the physical sensations that make up the experience of pain. They can be described on four dimensions: (1) location—where on your body the pain is experienced, (2) intensity—how intense the pain is, (3) quality—the nature of the sensations (e.g., dull, aching, sharp, burning, stabbing) and (4) time—how the sensations vary over time.

Emotional

This includes all of the emotional states that accompany the experience of pain as well as the effects of pain on your life. Examples include fear, anxiety, worry, depression, despair, guilt, anger, and irritability.

Mental

This includes awareness of pain, focus of attention, memory of pain and other experiences, expectations regarding the pain condition and your ability to cope with it, perceptions of ongoing life events, thoughts that accompany emotions, decision-making processes, attitudes toward yourself and others, etc. Another word for mental is *cognitive*.

Actions

This includes all the things that you actually do in response to the experience of pain, ongoing emotional states, and the consequences of pain on your life. It also includes physical activities that can affect your pain intensity as well as influence your thoughts and emotions.

Physical Environment

This includes all aspects of the physical environment that affect your awareness of pain or ability to cope with pain. Examples may include weather conditions, housing conditions, physical objects such as beds and chairs, material resources, means of transportation, etc.

Social Environment

This refers to individuals who can affect and are affected by your pain condition. It includes family and friends, medical care professionals, employers and co-workers, representatives of the disability compensation system, etc.

---

*It is important to understand that each of these factors cannot be considered in isolation. That is, each element interacts with and is affected by every other element.

Patients can then be given a list of factors that open and close the gate (cf. Philips, 1988). Modifying the list appearing in Turk et al. (1983), we suggest the following as self-management procedures that may help close the gate:

1. Physical factors
    a. Application of heat or cold.
    b. Massage.
    c. Transcutaneous electrical nerve stimulation (TENS).
    d. Stretching (range of motion) exercises.
2. Emotional factors
    a. Maintaining relative emotional stability by avoiding excess or inappropriate anger, depression, fear, and anxiety.
    b. Managing tension through rest breaks and time-out relaxation exercises.
    c. Positive emotions such as love and compassion, joy, humor and laughter, and optimism.
3. Mental factors
    a. Distraction of attention away from pain to other thoughts and activities.
    b. Increased involvement and interest in life activities and social interaction.
    c. Positive attitudes toward oneself, other people, and the future.
4. Actions
    a. Maintaining an appropriate physical activity level.
    b. Maintaining a good balance of work and recreational and social activities.
    c. Maintaining optimal physical health through regular physical exercise, healthy eating patterns, and refraining from unhealthy habits such as smoking and excess alcohol consumption.

Finally, mention is made of the endorphins since many chronic-pain patients have heard about them in the popular media. We begin by briefly mentioning the process of their discovery: Initially, scientists were interested in discovering how morphine and related narcotic substances could block pain. Eventually, they discovered the existence of specialized nerve cells that respond to morphine by blocking responsivity to pain. These nerve cells contain locks, and morphine serves as a key that turns the lock. Later, it was discovered that these specialized nerve cells do not exist in order to respond to morphine. Rather, the brain and spinal cord manufactures its own substance that is similar to morphine. These substances were named endorphins because they are *endo*genous (i.e., "internally generated") *morphine*-like substances. In reality, there are many specific forms of endorphin, and they play a role in other brain processes in addition to pain.

Of course, the primary question raised by pain patients is how is it possible to increase the availability of these endorphins. Responses to this question must be stated somewhat tentatively, since much is still unknown, and contradictory studies abound. First, we suggest that it would not be desirable to produce endorphins to such a degree that no pain could be felt. The same point is made with regard to closing the pain gate. It is important to be responsive to the warning function of acute pain. Second, we suggest that reliance on exogenous morphine-like substances (i.e., narcotic analgesics) may inhibit endorphin production, since the locks are already filled with keys, making endorphin production unnecessary. We then mention that there is some suggestive evidence that endorphins may be increased by physical exercise and positive beliefs, expectations, and emotional states.

REVIEW OF MAJOR SELF-MANAGEMENT GOALS

After introducing the biopsychosocial model of pain, we find it useful to present an overall perspective on some of the major goals to be addressed in our self-management training program. It is pointed out that some goals may apply more to some patients than others. Major goals include the following:

1. Improve ability to divert attention away from pain sensations through activities and mental techniques.
2. Improve overall physical condition through physical reconditioning exercises.
3. Learn how to increase and better modulate daily physical activities.
4. Learn ways to cope more effectively with episodes of intense pain without having to rely on narcotic analgesics.
5. Learn how to manage depression better.
6. Learn how to manage anger better and to behave more assertively.
7. Learn how to cope more effectively with tension, anxiety, stressful life demands, and interpersonal conflict.

After briefly explaining each goal, we solicit feedback from each group member regarding which of these goals, if any, are considered personally relevant. Almost invariably, each of the participants is able to list at least one of these goals. Most indicate that several, if not all, of these goals are important.

It is emphasized that none of these goals can be completely met while patients are in the pain program. In fact, many self-management goals are never considered fully accomplished and are instead viewed as life-long goals. As a person's chronic pain, general physical health, and other life conditions change, adjustments in these goals need to be made. The pain program can be viewed as a time to identify and establish healthy pain-management goals, learn new methods of working toward these goals, and make a significant start in pursuit of these goals.

Although the intensive training component of our program is time-limited, we make an effort to be flexible and adapt the program content to the needs of the members comprising a particular pain group. Although each of the general topic areas reviewed in the next four chapters is always covered with patients who go through our program, we may emphasize or deemphasize particular components depending on the interests and needs of the group. In this way we differ from more highly structured programs such as the one described by Philips (1988). The self-management program she describes consists of nine weekly outpatient sessions, each devoted to a specific topic. A program such as this is well suited for a very time-limited group approach, since it packs a maximum amount of information into a minimum period of time. It also allows for a more tightly controlled research evaluation, since it follows a very standardized procedure. Our preference is to maintain greater flexibility in the sequencing, pacing, and amount of time spent on particular self-management topics.

ESSENTIAL TARGETS FOR CHANGE

In addition to presenting and establishing general self-management goals, pain management specialists should attempt to identify the essential ingredients needed to alter the chronic-pain syndrome. Although at this point the essential ingredients for effective chronic-pain management are unknown, we have found useful some suggestions made by Barlow (1988) in his important book on anxiety disorders. In this book, he identifies the essential targets for change in any affective therapy aimed at treating emotional disorders, with special reference to fear and anxiety reduction. Even though chronic pain is not an affective disorder, one could argue that the emotional component is responsible for most of the maladaptive features of the chronic-pain syndrome. Consequently, we believe his therapy model has relevance to work with chronic-pain patients. The three essential targets that are identified include dysfunctional action tendencies, a sense of uncontrollability and unpredictability, and self-focused attention.

Action Tendencies

Action tendencies refer to basic tendencies to act or cope with negative affect. They are targeted in recognition of the fact that emotions are primarily action tendencies. Melzack and Torgerson (1971), in their three-component model of pain, list the motivational-affective dimension along with the sensory-discriminative and cognitive-evaluative dimensions. The motivational-affective component impels an organism in pain to act in a way that relieves the aversive stimulation. A primary action tendency associated with pain is to discontinue ongoing goal-directed activities and withdraw to safety. Physical withdrawal, rest, and immobility have important survival value for acute pain, but they can become highly maladaptive with chronic pain. Other action tendencies associated with chronic pain stem from the tendency to anticipate future increases in pain intensity. One consequence of this anticipation is the tendency to avoid engaging in physical activities that have previously been associated with increased pain. Another anticipatory action tendency is to be continuously "on guard" by tensing certain skeletal muscles or using protective movements and postures. Other action tendencies associated with the chronic-pain syndrome are repetitive attempts to seek medical treatment, including use of narcotic analgesics and requests for potentially risky surgical procedures.

Essential to Barlow's (1988) theory is that in order to treat certain emotional disorders effectively, these action tendencies must be prevented from occurring while the target emotion is being experienced. This relates to the fact that many of the treatments for phobias are based on exposure to fear-arousing stimuli. It is also interesting to note that Morita Therapy, a Japanese school of psychotherapy that has influenced our thinking, requires patients to meet their daily responsibilities and engage in productive behaviors *in spite of* the presence of inhibiting emotions such as anxiety and depression (Reynolds, 1976, 1984). In a similar manner, maladaptive action tendencies must be prevented and alternative coping behaviors must be utilized when patients are experiencing pain. It is during exposure to distressing emotions and pain that new learning can take place. Exposure and response-prevention methods for chronic pain can include the following:

1. Elimination of narcotic analgesics and other habit-forming central nervous system depressants.
2. Behavioral exposure, in gradual increments, to previously avoided physical activities.
3. Reduction of anticipatory action tendencies associated with guarded movements or excessive reliance on canes, crutches, and

other bracing devices through graded physical reconditioning exercises.

4. Reduction of anticipatory action tendencies associated with increased muscle tension through relaxation exercises or biofeedback training.

5. Substitution of healthy cognitive and behavioral coping responses during times of increased pain intensity. These may be naturally occurring episodes of pain exacerbations or artificially induced through standard laboratory pain-stimulation procedures (e.g., cold pressor task, tourniquet method to produce ischemic forearm pain).

6. The countering of social withdrawal by encouraging active participation in a group treatment program and increased interaction with family and friends.

7. Provision of positive social reinforcement for engaging in healthy, non-pain-related behaviors.

From this perspective, the goal is not to eliminate pain totally any more than the goal of affective therapies is to eliminate all negative emotions. The ability to experience pain, fear, sadness, and anger is not only essential to survival but is also an intrinsic part of human existence. To some observers, it is what adds meaning to life. On the other hand, maladaptive action tendencies arising from distortions or exaggerations of these fundamental experiences create problems and interfere with healthy living.

Sense of Control

Barlow (1988) suggests that at the core of the complex cognitive–affective structure of anxiety is a sense of uncontrollability and unpredictability. He also notes that uncontrollability or helplessness is a fundamental feature of depression. It should be readily apparent that uncontrollability and associated feelings of helplessness and hopelessness are significant components of the chronic-pain syndrome as well. Chronic pain can be viewed as a highly aversive experience over which the person has little or no control. In a recent study reported by Rudy, Kearns, and Turk (1988), it was found that perceived interference of pain and lack of self-control were the primary mediating links between pain and depressed mood. Crisson and Keefe (1988) found that chronic-pain patients who were more psychologically distressed and likely to use maladaptive pain-coping strategies were those who perceived outcomes as controlled by chance factors such as fate or luck. In other words, those who do not perceive themselves to be in control of life events are more likely to show negative features of the chronic-pain syndrome.

Consequently, another essential target for treatment of affective disorders as well as chronic-pain management is to increase the perception of control. In his summary on the issue of uncontrollability, Barlow (1988) states, "Even aversive events of substantial intensity or duration will be better tolerated (with marked individual differences) if they occur predictably and if the organism at least perceives that some control over these events is possible. Lack of predictability or controllability of these 'stressful' events seems to lead to chronic anxiety and/or depression" (p. 264). To chronic anxiety and depression, we would add the chronic-pain syndrome.

It is important to point out again that it is not the experience of pain, fear, and other distressing emotions per se that is problematic. It is the perception of unpredictability and uncontrollability over aversive events that creates problems. Barlow (1988) also notes that perceptions of mastery and control can reflect deeper cognitive structures or cognitive sets than are acquired earlier in development. We would also suggest that perceptions of control over pain can reflect earlier developmental experiences.

Nearly all of the techniques used in self-management training can be viewed as attempts to increase patients' perception of control over pain and its disruptive effects on their lives. It is in this respect that self-management approaches have the advantage over medical methods. Patients learn ways of controlling pain on their own instead of being the passive recipients of methods administered by a professional. Following the suggestion by Miller (1979), Barlow (1988) also notes that it may not even be control per se that is essential. The "illusion" or perception of control itself may be more important. This view is in accord with our frequent clinical observation that patients who clearly benefit from self-management training do not necessarily report less pain but, rather, an *increased sense of control over pain*. It also suggests that the effectiveness of specific pain-management techniques, such as relaxation exercises and training in cognitive coping strategies, is based not only on the intended effects but also on the extent to which they enhance perceptions of control. The importance of perceived control was demonstrated in a study using EMG biofeedback training for tension headache sufferers (Andrasik & Holroyd, 1980; Holroyd et al., 1984). By manipulating perceived success in reducing muscle tension through bogus feedback displays, they were able to show that patients who believed they were most successful reported the greatest reduction in headaches, irrespective of the actual EMG changes.

Self-Focused Attention

The final essential aspect of treatment is helping patients shift away from an excessive internal focus of attention to a more external focus. Barlow (1988) suggests that a significant component of pathological as opposed to "normal" anxiety is a persistent internal self-evaluative focus of attention. This internal focus results in increased emotional arousal, disruption in performance, and creation of a vicious cycle that he calls "anxious apprehension."

A very similar vicious cycle exists in many chronic-pain patients who become preoccupied with somatic sensations. Attention is not confined to the purely sensory aspects of pain but is also given to evaluations of the meaning of these sensations with regard to their well-being. In other words, this self-focus includes an important emotional component that can increase autonomic arousal, muscle tension, and eventually pain itself. As patients adopt an increasingly vigilant somatic focus, other body sensations are noticed, elaborated on, and sometimes misperceived as indications of further breakdowns in physical health. Thus, it is not uncommon for chronic-pain patients to report an entire array of somatic complaints in addition to their original pain complaint.

With increased internal focus, attention to the external environment decreases. With diminished awareness of social cues, chronic-pain patients appear self-centered, preoccupied with their own needs, and oblivious to the needs and feelings of others. Diminished awareness of task-related stimuli can interfere with the performance of many activities. Inactivity, social withdrawal, and depression all contribute to increased pain preoccupation.

Consequently, an essential goal of self-management training is to help patients shift their focus of attention to external stimuli. Increased participation in vocational or other meaningful work-related activities, enjoyable hobbies, and recreational activities can help divert attention away from pain. Increased participation in normal social activities where pain-related topics are not included as major topics of conversation is also essential. Efforts to increase the range of distracting activities are discussed in greater detail in Chapter 5.

SUMMARY

Those individuals who have developed a maladaptive chronic-pain syndrome are appropriate candidates for referral to an intensive multidisciplinary self-management program. Preparation for self-management should begin with the referring physician, who has determined that conventional medical/surgical procedures are no longer appropriate. Patients are accepted for self-management training only after a thorough biopsychosocial assessment. The primary initial goal of pain management is to help patients redefine their problem. This requires shifting from an acute, biomedical disease perspective to a multifaceted biopsychosocial perspective. Patients are introduced to this model by discussing interactions among five primary variables: pain sensations, emotions, cognitions, overt behavior, and socioenvironmental factors. Primary emphasis is placed on changing behavior and cognitions. To enhance the credibility of this perspective, patients are given a simple neurophysiological model that includes the gate-control theory, role of the endorphins, and multiple brain functions involved in pain. Major self-management goals are reviewed, after which patients are encouraged to identify their own specific goals. Drawn from Barlow's (1988) model for treatment of anxiety disorders, three essential targets for change are identified. These are to modify maladaptive action tendencies, to increase perception of control, and to reduce self-focused attention.

CHAPTER 4

Self-Management of Physical Activities

One of the major characteristics of chronic pain is its association with physical disability. Most individuals who are referred to our program report limitations in their physical capabilities as a result of their pain condition. Perhaps the most prominent aspect of disability for many is its effects on employment. The basis for the vast disability compensation system in this country is inability to engage in gainful employment. Besides employment, people with chronic pain report other significant functional limitations. In the broadest sense, functional limitation refers to the inability or difficulty in performing any purposeful function or activity as a result of pain, disease, or impairment. Although such functions may include perceptual and other cognitive tasks, our concern here is with physical functions and activities that are considered within the normal range of most people. Of greatest relevance to our chronic-pain patients are limitations in those physical activities that they previously performed before onset of their pain-related condition. These may include various recreational activities (e.g., tennis, golf, hiking, fishing, skiing, sailing, bowling, visiting friends, going to movies or sporting events), household chores (e.g., shopping, cooking, housecleaning, doing dishes, gardening, household repairs), sexual activities, and activities associated with employment.

Unfortunately, many chronic-pain patients view their limitations exclusively from a biomedical disease perspective. According to this perspective, physical limitations are directly and solely the result of pain and the pathophysiological factors causing the pain. Consequently, the only way to reduce or eliminate these limitations is to eliminate or cure the underlying pain condition. Since the patients are unable to achieve this cure, they are forced to be physically disabled. The biopsychosocial perspective recognizes that other factors contribute to disability besides the pain itself. These include deconditioning, fear, depression, environmental consequences, other intrapsychic payoffs, and the normal effects of aging.

FACTORS CONTRIBUTING
TO PHYSICAL LIMITATIONS

Through lectures and group discussion we attempt to help patients explore some factors that may be contributing to their physical limitations.
Eventually, we hope to help them identify concrete self-management
goals that may increase their physical capabilities and activity level as well
as reduce the negative impact of physical limitations on their lives. We
recognize that many forms of physical impairment associated with injury
or disease result in physical limitations. Some patients have developed
chronic-pain conditions following serious injuries that have resulted in
permanent damage to their limbs or back. Others may have suffered
injury as a result of repetitive unsuccessful surgical attempts to eliminate
their pain. Still others have physical impairment as a result of chronic
degenerative disease processes affecting their joints, vertebrae, nervous
system, or other body structures.

It must also be recognized that the natural aging process typically
imposes progressive limitations on physical strength, agility, and endurance. A 65-year-old person, even in the best of health, is not as physically
capable as most 25-year-olds. Even professional athletes, who earn their
living through their physical skills must eventually retire from active
competition, irrespective of how much they train or condition themselves.
Progressive limitation through aging is a fact of life.

Physical limitations that can be directly attributed to permanent
physical impairments or the aging process are to be considered true and
necessary physical limitations. Such limitations must ultimately be
accepted. A 55-year-old male with chronic low back pain unrelieved by
lumbar laminectomy and disk excision may have to accept the fact that he
should not attempt to work in a job that requires heavy lifting.

Unfortunately, many individuals with chronic pain are more limited
than necessary. Some have learned to respond to their pain condition with
greater physical disability than what may be attributed to their actual
organic impairment. Others develop additional physical limitations as a
result of the way in which they perceive and cope with their pain.

Deconditioning

One of the most common bases for excess disability is deconditioning as a
result of prolonged inactivity. Bortz (1984) refers to this as the "disuse
syndrome." Deconditioning or "getting out of shape" from disuse results
in decreased muscle tone and muscle atrophy, joint stiffening, bone
demineralization, and loss of aerobic fitness or cardiopulmonary endurance. Deconditioning is also commonly associated with weight gain and
excess body fat (obesity), depression, and premature aging (Bortz, 1984).

Deconditioning is an important component of the vicious cycle individuals with chronic pain often find themselves involved in. Sometimes, deconditioning and obesity contribute to the initial development of pain problems in locations such as the back. Irrespective of the cause, acute pain involving the back, neck, arms, and legs typically results in restricted activity. People automatically tend to decrease physical activity when specific movements, activities, and body positions result in increased pain. Standard medical treatment recommendations for many acute injuries and diseases are immobilization (e.g., splints, body casts, braces, and traction), bed rest, and restricted activity in order to facilitate the healing process. It is then expected that once the acute injury has healed or the disease has run its course, normal activities may be resumed. Obviously, this conventional wisdom is borne out in many instances. On the other hand, some are now questioning the value of bed rest for even acute cases of low back pain and sciatica (Waddell, 1987). A study by Deyo, Diehl, and Rosenthal (1986) found that 2 days of bed rest are as effective as 7 days and result in considerably less lost time from work.

Unfortunately, in the case of chronic pain, immobilization, rest, and inactivity are often prolonged, resulting in significant deconditioning. Prolonged immobilization and inactivity are other unfortunate consequences of applying the acute medical perspective to chronic pain. Referring to conventional treatment of low back pain, Waddell (1987) states, "there is strongly suggestive evidence that rest, particularly prolonged bed rest, may be the most harmful treatment ever devised and a potent cause of iatrogenic disability" (p. 640). Deconditioning leads to decreased pain and activity tolerance, thereby creating a vicious cycle. When inactive individuals are also obese, an increased load is placed on weight-bearing structures such as the back, hips, and legs. Unfortunately, since these areas are often associated with pain in the first place, the original pain can become exacerbated.

Fear

For many chronic-pain patients, fear plays a significant role in promoting excess disability. Specifically, patients report concerns that they will further injure themselves or significantly increase their pain by engaging in particular activities. Some patients go so far as to envision themselves confined to a wheel chair or permanently paralyzed if they exceed their physical limits. Patients with chronic back pain are especially prone to report these fears. Some attribute onset of their back pain to a relatively innocuous, routine activity such as bending, twisting, or lifting. In such instances, they may appraise the experience by saying to themselves, "my back just gave out," or "I felt it snap," or "something seemed to pop out of place." This implies that the back is quite vulnerable to mechanical breakdown with common physical activities.

Unfortunately, traditional medical views of back pain often contribute to unnecessary patient fears. In discussing what he considers to be medical mythology regarding back pain, Sarno (1984a) states, "one of the basic myths, fundamental to many others, is that the back is a delicate structure, to be protected carefully from strain or damage" (p. 42). Furthermore, in their effort to explain the etiology of recurrent back pain, physicians have often pointed to various specific structural defects in the spine. Confusion and anxiety may be created when patients are given different diagnoses and opinions by different physicians. Degenerative processes in particular are often suggested to be a major culprit behind back pain in spite of the lack of evidence relating the two. The very use of the term "degeneration" (e.g., degenerated lumbar disk) can be frightening to patients. Patients can easily imagine their spine as a progressively deteriorating, crumbling, fragile structure that may suddenly break if they make the wrong movement. This obviously evokes considerable fear of physical activity.

Sarno (1984a) reports that just explaining to patients that they have a relatively benign psychosomatic condition (that he calls the "tension myositis syndrome") is sometimes sufficient to alleviate patient anxiety. Also contributing to patient fears is the common medical advice that when he or she experiences episodes of more intense pain, he or she should rest in bed and refrain from all activity. This further contributes to the patient's idea that his back is so fragile that he may seriously injure himself if he engages in physical activity. When pain does subside with rest and inactivity, it is only natural for the patient to conclude that control over pain can only be maintained by greatly curtailing physical activities.

The consequence of this fear is twofold. First, it sets up a pattern of conditioned avoidance. Specific activities are avoided in the same way that a phobic avoids the feared object. The person is then locked in a vicious cycle whereby fear leads to avoidance and continued avoidance maintains the fear. Second, fear contributes to increased muscle tension that often increases pain intensity creating another vicious cycle.

Depression

Another factor contributing to inactivity, deconditioning, and excess disability is depression. Since depression often accompanies chronic pain, this may become another component in the vicious cycle of chronic pain and disability. Depression contributes to inactivity since part of the phenomenology of depression is a decreased energy, initiative, enthusiasm, and desire to engage in social and physical activities. Physical limitations, restricted activity, and avoidance of previously rewarding social and recreational activities contribute to more pain preoccupation, depression, low self-esteem, feelings of helplessness and hopelessness, etc.

Many use their pain as an excuse to avoid certain activities. For example, a spouse may suggest going out to visit some friends. The partner with chronic pain may respond by saying "I'm just not up to it tonight, my back is killing me." In this case, the partner may be using pain as an excuse to avoid social contact when the real reason is depression. Thus, we encourage our patients to be honest with themselves when they avoid specific physical activities. We ask whether the activity is avoided because the patient is truly unable to perform it without significantly increasing pain, or is it because he or she just doesn't "feel like doing it" (i.e., is feeling depressed). This distinction is important, since one of the recommended steps in managing depression, as discussed in Chapter 7, is to engage in previously rewarding activities in spite of the fact that one "does not feel like it."

Environmental Consequences

Environmental rewards for excess disability are well known and have been mentioned earlier. These include attention and sympathy from others, avoidance of unwanted activities and responsibilities, procurement of drugs, and financial compensation through personal injury suits, disability compensation, etc. Although we have no doubt that these "secondary gains" do contribute to chronic-pain behavior and excess disability, it is our impression that they do not play as significant a role as sometimes suggested by behavioral psychologists such as Fordyce (1976) and Roberts (1986).

Nevertheless, we do raise this issue with our patients. When first discussing environmental rewards ("pain payoffs") with patients, it is often necessary to proceed with some caution. Patients tend to resist the implication that they are using their disability or even exaggerating it in order to obtain some interpersonal or tangible reward. Thus, it is important to present this subject in such a way that it minimizes patient resistance. We begin by suggesting that these rewards apply to some people with chronic pain and that they might want to take an honest look at themselves to see if it applies to them in any way. It is also pointed out that the contribution of these pain payoffs to disability is not necessarily conscious and deliberate. For this reason, the ability to identify specific pain rewards may require considerable courage and soul searching. Patients are asked if they can think of an occasion upon which they used their pain, or any illness for that matter, to get out of doing something they did not want to do. This usually evokes some examples that can be used to stimulate further group discussion.

Much has also been made of the public disability compensation system for reinforcing inactivity and disability behavior and thereby discouraging return to work. This system includes state-run Worker's Compensation programs, two national programs administered by the Social Security Administration (Social Security Disability Insurance and Supplemental Security Income), and two programs administered by the Veterans Administration that are available only to veterans of the U.S. Military Service (service-connected compensation and non-service-connected pension benefits). In each of these programs, pain complaints alone are considered insufficient bases for awarding disability payments. Each program requires medically verified evidence of physical impairment when pain is involved. Unfortunately, medical determination of physical impairment and legal/administrative determination of disability are very complex issues subject to differences of opinion, inconsistencies, and subjective judgments (Osterweis et al., 1987).

Regarding medical determinations, it was emphasized earlier that many chronic-pain patients do not present clear, unequivocal, objective evidence of physiological abnormality. Thus, physicians must make their judgments on the basis of physical examination and patient reports that are subject to considerable manipulation by the pain patient. Applicants for disability benefits who do not present clear evidence of physical impairment may attempt to bolster their claim by exaggerating their functional limitations or reports of pain, muscle weakness, and sensory loss during the clinical examination. This may be especially likely for those with limited financial resources and job skills who anticipate difficulties in being awarded disability compensation or who have already been turned down and are in the process of appealing their claim. It is important to keep in mind that exaggerated presentations of functional impairment do not necessarily represent deliberate attempts to deceive physicians or disability rating boards.

Once disability compensation has been awarded, there may be little incentive to improve functional capabilities and seek vocational training or alternative employment, particularly if it is anticipated that these activities will result in loss of benefits. Those with the least incentive to improve their functional capabilities, return to work, and discontinue disability compensation are those who have few job skills, little education, a long period of unemployment, and little chance of reemployment because of age, poor medical history, and adverse economic conditions. Other reasons for maintaining an excessive level of disability and avoiding vocational rehabilitation are discussed in Chapter 9.

Although it is popular to criticize the disability compensation system and other entitlement programs for their tendency to discourage efforts to return to gainful employment, it is not our purpose to suggest changes in public policy. Rather, in our work with groups of individual pain patients, we attempt to help them establish specific realistic goals for minimizing their physical limitations and improving functional capabilities in a number of areas. This may involve return to work, or it may involve other volunteer, recreational, and social activities.

MODULATING PHYSICAL ACTIVITY

A general treatment goal in most chronic-pain management programs is to increase physical activity level and decrease exaggerated or excessive disability behavior. Although we agree with this general goal, we believe that emphasis should also be placed on modulation of physical activity. Although many chronic-pain patients are very inactive and spend excessive time reclining in bed or resting in a sitting position, many also tend to vacillate between underactivity and excessive overactivity. Excessive overactivity refers to any physical activity that results in a significant exacerbation of pain. We also refer to this as exceeding one's physical limits.

A common example is a person with chronic low back pain who experiences "good days" and "bad days." Good days occur when pain and muscle spasms are less intense, and the person feels relatively energetic and in a good mood. Bad days are the opposite: Pain and spasms are much more intense, and the person feels discouraged and incapable of any physical activity. As a result, narcotics are taken in larger quantities, and most of the day is spent in bed. Good days are then viewed as opportunities to be more active and accomplish various chores that have been neglected. Thus, on any given good day the person is likely to be much more physically active and, as a result, take on too much, "overdo it," and end up later that day or the next day in pain and misery. As this repetitive, vicious cycle is carried out over time, good days become more and more infrequent, and the person becomes increasingly fearful of attempting many physical activities. Examples such as this are readily acknowledged by many of our patients. We then point out that these swings in activity level can be prevented by regulating activity on a more consistent, daily basis through proper use of pacing and other procedures.

Activity modulation is actually one aspect of a much broader self-management theme that we emphasize throughout the program. This theme, which can be called lifestyle balance, stresses the importance of moderation and finding a middle ground between extremes. It has much in common with Marlatt's (1985) discussion of lifestyle balance as a means of preventing relapse among those with addictive disorders. For example, in working with problem drinkers, Marlatt (1985) emphasizes finding a balance between shoulds and wants in daily activities as well as avoiding the extremes of excessive restraint or overcontrol and excessive indulgence or undercontrol. With pain patients it is also important to emphasize balance between time spent in relaxation and physical activity as well as balance in how they go about engaging in physical activities.

In our program, self-management of daily physical activities is presented in three phases. First, we discuss ways of determining true physical limitations as opposed to excessive disability. Second, we discuss basic self-management principles for modulating physical activity on a daily basis (e.g., use of proper body mechanics and pacing procedures). Finally, the issue of self-acceptance in spite of having physical limitations is addressed.

DISCOVERING TRUE PHYSICAL LIMITATIONS

We begin by making a hypothetical distinction between true and apparent physical limitations and/or capabilities. Physical limitations and capabilities, as applied to many chronic-pain patients, may refer to basic physical capacities such as sitting tolerance, distance walked, or amount of weight that can be lifted. They can also refer to any number of specific functional activities of relevance to the patient such as gardening, vacuuming one's carpet, sewing, typing, pruning trees, playing golf, backpacking, etc. True limitations are necessitated by one's age and the presence of irreparable physical damage (to the neuromuscular system). True physical capabilities refer to one's potential. Apparent physical limitations and capabilities refer to the patient's current level of functioning. Implicit in this distinction is the idea that most pain-program participants are currently functioning at a level that is below their potential. At the same time, we recognize that the majority of our patients do have some legitimate physical limitations relating to their pain condition, although for some these may be minimal.

The gradual accumulation of excess disability is presented as a very common, naturally occurring process as the chronic-pain syndrome develops and continues over many years. To be avoided are any implications that the patient is being weak, lazy, or manipulative. Using our lecture/group discussion format, we review each of the factors contributing to excessive disability including deconditioning, depression, fear/avoidance, and disability payoffs. Each of these factors is subject to modification through self-management training and practice.

The process of discovering true physical limitations involves a number of components, including initiating a physical reconditioning program, discontinuing use of narcotic analgesics, eliminating rewards for disability behavior (or increasing incentives for healthy, physical activity), and making appropriate use of trial-and-error learning. Although patients agree to physical exercise and narcotic reduction prior to entering the program, the rationale for these procedures can be made more explicit in the context of reducing excess disability.

INITIATING A PHYSICAL RECONDITIONING PROGRAM

Physical reconditioning is a major goal for the vast majority of our patients, especially those who have become very inactive as a result of back and other musculoskeletal pain conditions. Irrespective of the specific pain condition, initiation and maintenance of an active exercise program are essential components of our self-management program. Many patients are initially reluctant to engage in physical reconditioning because of the expectation that it will elicit increased pain. Thus, it is important that they be given a clear and reasonable rationale for its value. When introducing the concept of physical exercise, an attempt should be made to avoid placing too much emphasis on its value as a specific pain-reduction technique. Some patients report reduction in pain intensity after establishing an exercise program, whereas others do not. In order for exercise to be of value, it is not necessary that it have a beneficial effect on specific physical problems assumed to be responsible for the pain. Instead, emphasis is placed on incorporating regular exercise into one's lifestyle. This differs from traditional rehabilitation philosophy, which views therapeutic exercise as a time-limited treatment measure that may be discontinued after rehabilitation is completed. We regard exercise as having more general value with respect to the patient's entire physical and psychological well-being.

Physical exercise has several potential benefits. First, it is expected that many patients will be able to increase their level of physical activity without a corresponding increase in pain intensity. In other words, we hope to decrease excessive physical limitations caused by deconditioning. Along with increases in general activity level, patients also begin to discover that they are able to engage in specific rewarding, pleasurable activities that have been discontinued because of preoccupation with pain and misery. Consequently, physical exercise and increased physical activity can serve to counteract depression. Exercise is also useful for managing stress and relieving tension arising from efforts to cope with chronic pain and other demands of everyday life. In short, we make it clear that physical exercise has both physical and psychological benefits. Rather than viewing their bodies solely as sources of discomfort and physical limitation, patients begin to develop a more positive perception of their physical well-being and increased confidence in their physical capabilities.

Three target areas for improvement are increasing joint flexibility, muscle tone, and aerobic fitness. Another important area of concern is body weight and percentage of body fat. It is now well known that the normal physiological consequences of prolonged immobilization and inactivity are decreased range of joint motion, decreased muscle strength, and reductions in cardiopulmonary efficiency and endurance.

In order to increase joint flexibility, patients are taught several specific stretching exercises. Considerable attention is given to flexibility of the neck and trunk. Neck mobility can be increased through forward flexion, side leaning, and rotation exercises. Back flexion exercises are used to increase flexibility of the trunk, which becomes limited as a result of low back pain. Examples include knee-to-chest, pelvic tilt, arching the back while kneeling (cat back), bending forward while sitting, floor touch, hamstring stretches, etc. Back extension exercises may also be of value, even for those with low back pain (Sarno, 1984b). Other specific stretching exercises may be prescribed for the shoulders and other joints depending on specific areas of limited movement. One major prerequisite to performing these exercises is that the patient should be relaxed since tense muscles work against the stretching process. A significant advantage of these exercises is that they can easily be done at home and require no special equipment.

Patients are also instructed in various muscle strengthening or toning exercises. Particular attention is given to muscles in the neck, shoulders and arms, back, abdomen, and legs. Muscles can be strengthened by lifting against gravity as well as by various isometric (static resistance) exercises. Preferable to most exercises, however, are isotonic (moving against resistance) ones that utilize weights (e.g., barbells and dumbbells) or special equipment comprised of weights and pulleys found in most gymnasiums and health clubs.

Finally, patients are encouraged to engage in exercises aimed at increasing aerobic fitness or cardiopulmonary endurance. Care must be taken to find exercises that do not exacerbate the pain condition. Although jogging may be an excellent aerobic exercise, very few of our patients are able to do this. Alternative aerobic exercises include riding a stationary bicycle, swimming, and brisk walking.

Detailed descriptions of specific physical exercises for specific pain conditions are beyond the scope of this book. There are a number of important principles that should be adhered to when one is instructing patients in a physical reconditioning program.

Baseline Assessment

A thorough baseline assessment is essential prior to initiating a physical reconditioning program. This assessment is used as a basis for developing a specific exercise program as well as a reference point to evaluate progress. Specific tests are available to assess each of the major target areas. Joint flexibility is assessed through standard range-of-motion tests (American Academy of Orthopaedic Surgeons, 1965). Methods for manually assessing muscle function are described by Daniels and Worthingham (1986) and Kendall (1983). An estimate of aerobic fitness can be obtained by taking pulse readings before, during, and after a prescribed period of aerobic activity such as pedaling on a stationary bicycle. More sophisticated evaluation procedures are described in Hojnacki and Halfman-Franey (1985) and Jones and Campbell (1982). Baseline assessment should also include body weight and an estimate of percentage of body fat.

Individualized Program

Based on the initial assessment, each patient is given a specific exercise prescription. This includes identifying concrete goals and specific exercises aimed at attaining these goals. For example, baseline assessment may indicate that a patient's forward trunk flexion while standing is 20 inches from the fingertips to the floor. A goal might be to increase flexion to the point where the patient can touch the floor. Specific flexibility exercises are then prescribed to enable the patient to eventually reach this goal. Each exercise is demonstrated, and then the patient is guided through the exercise to make sure it is done correctly. Each exercise prescription must be very specific and include references, as appropriate, to the correct body position, number of repetitions, duration of the exercise, speed of movement, amount of weight to be used, etc. When possible, it is especially important to develop functional goals in addition to specific exercise goals. Common functional goals include increasing distance walked or sitting time.

Initiation Phase

As previously mentioned, it is important that patients be given a thorough rationale for pursuing physical reconditioning. Many chronic-pain patients associate physical activity with pain and are resistant to performing activities perceived to increase their pain. Additionally, many patients have been advised by a physician to curtail specific activities or movements. Often such advice was given during the acute stage of the pain problem, when activity restriction may have been more appropriate. Thus, it is important to discuss patient's expectations of an exercise program to clear up misconceptions and identify realistic goals.

During the initial phase of a reconditioning program, patients are closely monitored, and the therapist assumes responsibility for setting the pace of each exercise. One of the most common problems in initiating an exercise program is the patients' tendency to exceed their limits by overdoing an exercise to the point where it results in a significant increase in pain. As a result, patients get discouraged and attempt to discontinue exercise altogether.

> For example, C.D. was a 37-year-old male patient with chronic left leg pain following a motorcycle accident 12 years earlier. Although he had engaged in regular body-building exercises prior to his injury, he was overweight and "out of shape" when he entered our program. When our kinesiotherapist first introduced the patients to the weight equipment in the gym, C.D. paid little attention and immediately began demonstrating to the other patients the amount of weight he could lift. It was not surprising that he reported a significant increase in his pain the following morning along with a desire to leave the program. Although he initially denied that his behavior in the gym had anything to do with his increased pain, he was persuaded to remain in the program.

With patients such as C.D., our therapists place considerable emphasis on slow and gradual progress. Patients must be repeatedly cautioned against exercising to their pain tolerance level. To prevent this from occurring, Fordyce (1976) recommends that therapists set limits for each exercise below the level where the patient would experience pain. Sternbach (1987) suggests a limit of one-third of the pain tolerance level as a starting point, assuming a twice-daily exercise program.

Although it is ideal during the initial phase to supervise each patient closely, this becomes more difficult in group programs such as ours. Group exercise can be more economical in terms of staff time and certainly more enjoyable for the participants. However, it becomes more difficult to monitor each patient closely since the therapist must circulate among them. Patients must also be repeatedly reminded that they should avoid the temptation to compete with one another, since each has his or her own individual goals. This warning is especially critical when one is working with those patients who have learned to associate competition with physical exercise.

Monitoring and Reinforcing Progress

Rather than compete with one another, patients can compete with themselves by measuring their own progress against their initial baseline. Thus, it is very useful to have them record progress in each exercise and even graphically display their progress. This can serve as a basis for both self-reinforcement and praise from staff. Throughout the reconditioning program, it is important that staff attend to and reinforce indications of progress. Displays of pain behavior when patients are performing these exercises are ignored. As exercise behavior is observed, therapists can obtain many clues regarding the patient's approach to physical activity in general. For example, some appear hesitant and must be encouraged or pushed, whereas others seem to show reckless disregard and must be repeatedly restrained from overdoing each exercise.

Maintenance

All physical exercise programs will be unproductive if they are discontinued after a few weeks or months. In hospital-based pain programs such as ours, there is a tendency for some participants to stop exercising shortly after being discharged. Thus, the necessity of long-term maintenance must be emphasized from the very beginning. Toward the end of the hospital phase, each patient should be required to develop a specific home exercise program. In outpatient programs home exercise prescriptions are developed from the beginning. Unfortunately, there is considerable evidence that the majority of people in general discontinue an exercise program within 6 months of beginning it (Dishman, 1982). Maintenance may be facilitated if patients are given increased responsibility for performing their exercises during the active treatment phase and if the problem of maintenance is discussed directly with them. Patients are encouraged to identify potential obstacles to maintenance and discuss what might be done about them. It is recommended that they develop maintenance enhancement strategies such as exercising with others, continuing to keep records of progress, alternating exercises to reduce boredom, and choosing exercises that tend to be fun and intrinsically rewarding. Although many exercises can be performed at home, we encourage use of community facilities that contain swimming pools, stationary bicycles, and other special exercise equipment.

REDUCE OR ELIMINATE NARCOTIC USE

In order for chronic-pain patients to discover their true physical limitations, it is necessary for them to be able to perceive pain sensations. Use of narcotic analgesics serves to dull or mask these sensory signals, thereby setting the stage for abuse of limits and possible excessive wear on already damaged body structures. Thus, reduction and total elimination of narcotic use are considered to be additional requirements for determining true physical limitations.

Most of our patients are willing to accept this rationale as reason enough to reduce or eliminate their use of narcotic analgesics. There are those, however, who strongly resist this idea, claiming that narcotics are essential to maintain their desired physical activity level. Some view their pain as being so disabling that they would be incapable of doing any meaningful physical activity without the regular use of narcotics. Others report using narcotics only when they intend to engage in a specific physical activity that otherwise would be prohibitive because of extreme pain. Many physicians also consider this a valid basis for prescription of narcotics, especially if there is clear evidence indicating an organic basis for the pain.

Although admission to our inpatient program requires patient willingness to be tapered from narcotic use, we recognize that, ultimately, the decision to use or refrain from narcotics rests with the patient. Thus, it is necessary to discuss this issue directly and openly with them rather to attempt to impose our values or coerce them into discontinuing all narcotic use. Strategies for dealing with patients who are resistant or ambivalent about giving up narcotics are discussed at greater length in Chapter 6.

DISCOVERING LIMITATIONS THROUGH TRIAL AND ERROR

As patients work on improving their general physical condition, eliminate narcotic use, and come to grips with any emotional and environmental reward factors that contribute to excess disability, they are still left with the task of determining their true physical capabilities and limitations. According to the biomedical model, specification of physical limitations is often the prerogative of physicians based on an analysis of the patient's "objective" medical status. In accordance with this model, the disability compensation system often asks physicians to make objective determinations regarding the pain patient's physical capabilities and limitations (e.g., "the patient should avoid lifting anything over 20 pounds").

The self-management perspective, on the other hand, places primary responsibility for determining limitations on the person with chronic pain. This is usually accomplished through a trial-and-error process over time. By attempting specific physical activities in a graded manner and attending to consequent pain feedback, the patient gradually learns which activities are within limits. It is important to emphasize that activities should be attempted in a gradual manner rather than in a pattern that requires considerably more exertion and effort than has been engaged in recently.

The process of discovering specific capabilities and limitations can be facilitated if the patient is given accurate information regarding his or her condition and support from rehabilitation specialists including physicians, nurses, and physical therapists. As discussed earlier, some pain patients have inaccurate perceptions of their physical conditions and see themselves as being more fragile than they actually are. A similar situation is found among some patients who, after a major coronary event, are afraid to engage in physical activity out of fear that they may trigger another heart attack. Such pain patients may need to be reassured by their physician that they will not suffer further damage by engaging in reasonable physical activity. They may also be told that the occurrence of pain does not necessarily indicate that their spine is in danger of breaking or their nerves becoming permanently damaged.

ACTIVITY MODULATION

During the process of discovering true physical limitations, the patient is reminded that it is also important to consider how one goes about performing specific activities. Many individuals with chronic pain stop engaging in certain activities that could be continued if they were to modify the manner in which these are performed. Consequently, we review several principles that should be adhered to when one engages in various activities including household chores, work-related responsibilities, and recreational activities.

Body Mechanics

Attention must be given to the way in which the body is used in performing physical activities. Since many of our patients have chronic back pain, particular attention is given to the way in which they use their backs when lifting, pushing, and pulling heavy objects. Since it is generally thought that improper lifting can contribute to the development of back pain, it is essential that patients be given instruction in proper lifting techniques such as:

1. Bend at the knees rather than at the waist.
2. Lift with the legs while making sure that the feet are firmly planted.

3. Keep the load close to the body.
4. Lift objects only chest high.
5. Avoid twisting when lifting.

Other principles that should be adhered to include making use of mechanical aids (e.g., hand truck, wheelbarrow, pushcart), splitting heavy loads into smaller loads, when possible pushing rather than pulling heavy loads, asking for help, etc. Since carelessness and hurry often lead to improper body mechanics, patients should be reminded to think jobs through prior to actually doing them.

Posture

Closely related to body mechanics during the performance of physical work is attention to posture during prolonged activities or tasks. Activities that require prolonged standing, walking, sitting, or driving can result in problems. Standing with one foot resting on a low stool, changing positions often, avoiding high-heeled or platform shoes when standing or walking for long periods, avoiding a slumping position when sitting, moving the car seat forward in order to keep the knees bent and higher than the hips when driving, and avoiding leaning forward for extended periods are examples of proper postural techniques.

In multidisciplinary treatment programs, it is important that the entire team (not just the physical and occupational therapists) be familiar with and use good body mechanics and posture. In addition to consistent modeling, this can help provide more consistent feedback to patients for following or not following these principles. Patients are reminded that knowing what the principles are and actually putting them into practice are two separate matters. The key, of course, is repetition to the point that safe practices become habitual.

One important activity that may require special attention is sex. Although patients are often hesitant to initiate the subject, many will admit, when asked, that their pain condition has significantly interfered with their sexual activities. Some admit to having discontinued sex altogether. It is recognized that sexual dysfunction can have many causes other than pain, including marital problems, depression, performance anxiety, abuse of alcohol and drugs, certain prescribed medications (e.g., antihypertensive medications), and some chronic diseases such as diabetes. Consequently, it may be necessary to do a more thorough biopsychosocial assessment when patients report sexual problems. When it is determined that sexual problems arise as a result of pain in an otherwise healthy relationship, it is important to explore with the patient (and partner) positions and body mechanics that may reduce the amount of pain experienced during intercourse. Those with chronic back pain may find useful the information presented in a chapter by White (1983) in his popular book *Your Aching Back*.

Physical Environmental Supports

Attention should also be given to proper arrangement of the physical environment to support proper body mechanics and posture. Those with chronic back pain should be concerned with choice of mattresses and seats to avoid aggravating their condition. Guidelines written for patients are also found in White's (1983) book. Those with shoulder and arm conditions may need to rearrange their home or work environment to facilitate easy reach of commonly used objects.

Pacing Procedures

Another important issue to discuss with patients is how they pace themselves when engaging in various physical activities. Many attempt to continue doing certain activities at the same pace as they did before the onset of their pain condition. As a result, they often experience an acute exacerbation of pain, become discouraged, and sometimes abandon the activity altogether. Some also use this as an excuse to use narcotics. Often, exacerbation of pain can be prevented by the patient's taking appropriate rest breaks or performing the task at a slower speed.

The appropriate use of rest breaks needs to be emphasized, since many individuals continue to engage in physical tasks until pain sensations force them to stop. By this time it is too late. Instead, patients should stop before pain increases. For example, if a patient experiences a significant increase in pain after sitting at a work bench for 2 hours, he should take a break after an hour and a half or so. Knowing when to stop results from a trial-and-error process over time.

Many patients are aware of their need to apply pacing procedures but have difficulty putting these into practice. One common obstacle is the tendency to become so engrossed in a particular task that patients forget to take a break. For example, a patient with chronic back pain may be working over the hood of an automobile in a way that requires the back to be in a flexed-forward position. While one is engaged in this activity, full attention is given to the task at hand, and there is no awareness of pain until the person attempts to straighten up. More effective self-management requires the person to find signals or reminders to take periodic breaks before it is too late. This may involve placing a clock in view, using kitchen timers, or breaking a larger job into smaller components (e.g., vacuuming one room at a time, mowing a lawn in sections).

In addition to knowing when to stop and take a break, it is important to consider the length of the break and what to do during the break. In order to make good use of a rest break, it is important that the person change position or body posture and engage in a relaxing activity that diverts attention to something else. As Sternbach (1987) succinctly tells his patients, "move your muscles and change your thoughts." Breaks are also good opportunities to make use of time-out relaxation techniques (see Chapter 7). The amount of time out before returning to the task may also need to be determined on a trial-and-error basis.

One objection raised by some patients is that they are not always able to apply pacing procedures. Most often this is heard from individuals who are considering return to employment (e.g., "no one would hire me if I had to take rest breaks," or, "there's no way I could keep a job if I had to pace myself"). Employment is only one of several areas where activity pacing applies, and such pacing often points out the necessity of choosing employment activities within one's physical limitations. Self-employment is another alternative that may allow greater flexibility. Irrespective of the specific physical activity, patients need to make use of good problem-solving skills in making effective use of pacing procedures.

Asking for Help and Saying "No"

Another common obstacle to applying effective activity modulation is refusal to ask for help when needed or failure to say "no" to a request that will likely aggravate a pain condition. Most patients can readily identify specific situations in which they attempted to perform a demanding physical task on their own and then paid the personal price of increased pain. We then try to elicit various self-statements that can serve as excuses to avoid seeking help. The following are some common examples:

"I don't like to bother other people."
"I don't want others to think I'm lazy."
"I don't want to pay someone else to do something I used to do on my own."
"I can't afford to hire someone else."
"I don't like being dependent on other people."

Each of these excuses can be discussed and challenged in a group setting. A similar procedure is used concerning situations in which other individuals ask the pain patient for help in performing a physical task. A case example we often use is that of a young male patient with chronic low back pain who successfully graduated from our program, returned home, and then months later responded to a request from his next door neighbor to help move a heavy portable spa. As a result, the patient suffered an acute back strain and was hospitalized, placed back on narcotics, and eventually readmitted to our program. This individual paid a considerable price for failing to say "no" to his neighbor's request. Negative self-statements associated with refusing such requests should be elicited, discussed, and challenged. In the case of the patient just mentioned, he informed us that since the neighbor had done favors for him in the past, he felt it was only fair that he return the favor. He did not want the neighbor to think badly of him. Other members of the group challenged his thinking by pointing out that he could have refused the request, given a reasonable explanation, and offered to help the neighbor in other ways.

SELF-ACCEPTANCE

A major underlying issue pertaining to difficulties in modulating daily physical activities is self-acceptance. We have found that one of the most difficult challenges facing many of our patients is learning how better to accept themselves in spite of having physical limitations. Although self-acceptance is a very nebulous concept, it is used as a topic for individual and group counseling. We have found it particularly useful to raise this issue for discussion in groups that have already established some cohesiveness and perceived mutual support.

Physical skills and capabilities comprise a major component of self-identity. In some cases, unique and special skills acquired as a result of native talent, special training, or persistent effort become bases for admiration from others as well as for personal pride and self-esteem. When the ability to engage in these skills is impaired as a result of a painful injury or disease, the result can be a significant blow to one's self-worth. In addition, there are many common physical skills and activities that are taken for granted by most healthy people. Walking, running, jumping, bending, pushing, pulling, and lifting, for example, may be ordinary, everyday actions. Although they are not used as a basis for pride and self-respect, they become a part of one's assumed identity. Little attention is given to these activities until some injury or disease makes it difficult or impossible to carry them out. When physical impairment from an injury or disease is long term, one is forced to go through a process of adaptation and redefinition of one's basic self-identity.

Individuals with chronic-pain conditions tend to have personal standards of reference by which they judge and evaluate their current physical condition and capabilities. Often these reference points consist of times in their life prior to their pain condition. To make this more clear, we ask our patients to think back to the time in their life when they considered themselves the most healthy and physically fit. Typically, they refer to some time between their late teens and early 30s. We then ask them to evaluate their current self-worth with respect to this earlier time. As a result of this process, many negative self-references tend to be elicited. These self-depreciatory perceptions can then be discussed and challenged by other group members.

In our experience, those who have difficulty accepting their current physical limitations respond in one of the following basic ways. Some become very depressed and physically inactive.

> For example, E.F. had been a high school athlete before suffering a serious knee injury in his early 20s. In time the injury healed, and he was able to resume normal activities. E.F. enjoyed jogging and basketball and eventually began to compete in marathon races, as well as play full-court basketball with a group of friends. These activities unfortunately aggravated his original injury to the point where he was unable to run without severe pain. His physician, of course, told him that he could no longer engage in these strenuous activities. Consequently, E.F. discontinued all forms of physical exercise and became very inactive, out of condition, and depressed. When it was pointed out that there were still many physical activities that he could do as long as he did them in moderation, he responded by saying to himself, "what's the use, why bother doing anything if you can't compete anymore?" His ideal standard of reference were athletes who must push themselves to their physical limits in order to succeed. Since he considered himself unable to meet this standard, he felt worthless and lost interest in all physical activities.

Another common response to difficulties in accepting physical limits is chronic frustration and irritability. Patients who experience these feelings often appear angry, and may present difficulties in getting along with other people. Each time they encounter a specific situation in which they are unable to perform an activity that they previously had done without effort (e.g., a household chore), they become frustrated and irritated with themselves. Often the muscle tension associated with this frustration only serves to increase pain intensity. Some even develop secondary pains such as tension headaches.

A third common pattern is the alternating cycle between overactivity and underactivity. Overactivity in this context stems from an effort to deny one's physical limitations and thus maintain a level of activity that existed prior to the onset of the pain condition. When this occurs, the result is increased pain that greatly increases the likelihood that the patient will resort to narcotic analgesics in an effort to maintain the desired activity level. Eventually, the person may find himself in such excruciating pain that he gives up all activity and resorts to bed rest. After a back operation, another one of our patients attempted to resume a level of strenuous physical activity that he enjoyed before the onset of his low back pain. As pain increased, he returned to his surgeon, who ended up recommending additional surgery. Following a period of forced inactivity and convalescence, the patient again attempted to pick up where he had left off. In spite of assistance from narcotics, the patient again began experiencing increased pain and consulted another surgeon who performed a third back operation. This cycle was repeated until, after the fifth operation, the patient sought admission to our chronic-pain management program.

It is important that we help patients understand how each of these patterns results in a self-defeating vicious cycle that serves to perpetuate increased pain and disability. Those who fall into the first pattern of depression and inactivity must learn alternative ways of evaluating themselves. This may involve identifying and challenging specific depressive cognitions (see Chapter 7). It also may entail changing their focus of attention from things that they can no longer do to things they still can do. This is much easier to accomplish if the patient can be taught or encouraged to seek new, self-reinforcing physical activities that can provide a sense of accomplishment. Hobbies and recreational activities can serve this purpose.

Besides encouraging rewarding physical activities, we attempt to challenge beliefs that equate personal worth with physical activities and accomplishments. This may involve considering the concept of intrinsic worth as opposed to worth that must be earned and achieved, or the idea that it is not only what you do that is important but what kind of person you are. Showing genuine interest in others, participating in various groups and organizations, or pursuing aesthetic, philosophical, religious, and other transcendent values are all ways of enhancing one's sense of worth and well-being apart from physical achievement.

Difficulties with self-acceptance among those who are chronically frustrated or trapped in the alternating pattern of overactivity and underactivity must also be discussed. These individuals have problems accepting their limitations and thus keep pushing themselves to achieve an activity level that they were able to maintain in the past. In group discussions we ask our patients, "What does it mean for you to give up doing certain activities or change the way you go about doing certain activities?" This often elicits important issues regarding pride and self-respect, acceptance by other people, masculine and feminine role identity, autonomy versus dependence, etc. Some of our patients equate realistic acceptance of physical limitations with giving up and accepting defeat. Such beliefs need to be challenged.

We also attempt to relativize the issue of physical limitations by suggesting that ultimately it must be faced by everybody, irrespective of whether one has a chronic-pain condition. Everyone has some physical limitations, and everyone develops more limitations as he or she grows older. Thus, it is not the fact of having limitations that is at issue; rather it is the perception of those limitations in terms of how they affect one's sense of well-being and worth.

Finally, the issue of acceptance is not a static, one-time event but is, rather, an ongoing process that continues throughout life. Growing older and confronting situations that can no longer be managed through previously learned physical skills force one continuously to adapt. This issue is especially salient for most of our elderly patients, some of whom were able to successfully self-manage their chronic pain for 40 or more years until they reached the time of retirement from work or experienced the death of a spouse or were stricken with a major illness. Sometimes the pain they thought they had learned to live with grew intolerable and incapacitating even though there had been no corresponding change in the medical condition considered responsible for the pain in the first place. As life situations and events change, so does everyone's physical status, all of which place new demands on coping capacities. These issues are all important topics for group discussion and individual counseling.

SUMMARY

The vast majority of people treated in chronic-pain programs present varying degrees of physical limitations related to their chronic-pain condition. Those who have developed many features of the chronic-pain syndrome typically present disability in excess of what their physical condition actually warrants. Excess disability behaviors may be attributed to the effects of deconditioning, depressed mood, a pattern of fear and learned avoidance, rewarding environmental consequences, and other personal payoffs. Our self-management approach to physical activity includes three phases. First, patients are taught to distinguish between apparent and true physical limitations and capabilities. True, or necessary, physical limitations are discovered by first reducing or eliminating factors contributing to excess disability. Emphasis in this chapter is placed on establishing and maintaining an individualized physical exercise program. In addition to reversing the effects of deconditioning, physical exercise has several psychological benefits as well. Second, patients are taught methods aimed at better modulating the way in which they go about performing various physical tasks. Attention to posture and proper body mechanics, use of environmental supports (physical and social), and application of pacing procedures are emphasized. Finally, we address the issue of self-acceptance in relationship to physical capabilities. Dysfunctional attitudes and beliefs are to be identified and replaced with more healthy, adaptive ones. A more positive self-appraisal can develop as the person discovers a wide variety of rewarding and constructive activities. Emphasis is placed on living a full and productive life in spite of the existence of physical impairment.

CHAPTER 5

Coping with Pain
through Distraction

Intrinsic to the nature of pain is its tendency to captivate our awareness. In order for pain to serve a useful warning function, it must interrupt ongoing attention. Survival depends on the ability to recognize acute pain signals quickly. This allows one to act appropriately to minimize bodily damage and do whatever is necessary to enable healing to take place. Ongoing activities are interrupted, enabling one to attend more fully to the overriding goal of seeking pain relief. However, there are some situations when acute pain must be ignored in order to accomplish some other, more important activity or goal. There are numerous accounts of individuals who have done heroic deeds, accomplished incredible feats, and pushed their endurance beyond normal limits in spite of having suffered a significant bodily injury. This points to a fundamental and somewhat paradoxical characteristic of pain. Pain is a powerful signal that tends to grab one's attention, yet pain can also be ignored. Given the right circumstances, even pain associated with serious injury or disease can be ignored.

Chronic, continuous pain may also dominate awareness even though it usually no longer serves a useful biological warning function. Instead, it tends to play a primarily disruptive role, diverting attention away from ongoing events and activities. Chronic pain also interferes with many forms of cognitive activity including memory, judgment, and problem-solving capabilities. Nevertheless, it is known that chronic pain can also be ignored. In fact, apart from drugs, the single most common means of coping with chronic pain down through the ages has probably been to divert attention away from it.

It is essential that patients undergoing self-management training understand the importance of distraction. Most are already aware to some degree of its value. However, for some, it may first be necessary to address resistance to the idea that distraction can be a useful coping strategy. Some object because of the erroneous assumption that if they acknowledge their ability to be distracted from pain, this would mean that their pain is less valid or objectively based. Unfortunately, this misconception can also be held by health care professionals. According to this idea, if a patient can be distracted from pain, it must mean that the pain is not very intense or as severe as the patient says it is (McCaffery, 1979). This misconception is usually based on a naive, dualistic assumption that in order for pain to have a physical (i.e., "real") basis, it cannot be influenced or overridden by mental activity.

This assumption is usually easy to dispel during the introductory presentation of the biopsychosocial model. It is pointed out that attention is always involved in pain perception and that sensory awareness does not directly and passively reflect bodily injury. A few simple examples can serve to illustrate this point. We ask our patients to imagine that they are viewing a very interesting or exciting program on television and that their pain intensity is at a mild or moderate level. Most patients are willing to admit that it is quite possible for them temporarily to "forget their pain" while absorbed in the program. We then ask what would happen if someone approached them during the viewing of this program and asked, "Do you have any pain?" Of course the answer would be "yes" since the question itself would immediately lead them to switch their attention from the television program to their own bodies. We further ask whether their bodies had healed during the time their attention was on the program and they were not aware of pain. In this case the answer is an obvious "no." The actual physical condition of the body and awareness of pain are not necessarily related.

Once this misconception is clarified, patients are almost always willing to admit that there are times when they become distracted away from their pain. Some object, however, to the use of distraction because it has only temporary value. When a period of distraction ends, pain awareness returns. This objection is based on a misunderstanding of the basic role of self-management. In a sense, all self-management techniques are temporary, but then so are pain medications. Although a cure may be desired, a more realistic objective is to cope with pain on a day-by-day or even moment-by-moment basis. Even though pain seems to return after one has been distracted, the alternative of continuous pain awareness is hardly preferable.

Another objection to the value of distraction is that it is ineffective when pain is at a high level of intensity. We agree that it is more difficult to use distraction when pain is intense. Nevertheless, the point should be made that it is possible to become distracted away from even severe pain, especially in emergency situations. To illustrate this point, we relate an experience reported by one of our former patients.

One day, G.H., who suffered from chronic low back pain, was home alone and lying in bed. He had exceeded his physical limitations the previous day and was now experiencing a significant flare-up in pain intensity. As he lay in bed, he felt totally miserable and unable to get up. His preoccupation with pain and disability was interrupted by the sound of someone ringing the doorbell and pounding on his front door. Although he initially ignored this intrusion, hoping the person would go away, he eventually hobbled out of bed to find out what was going on. He opened the door to a neighbor who excitedly informed him that smoke and flames were coming out of a corner of his roof. Suddenly, G.H. forgot his back pain. After making sure the fire department had been called, he grabbed a ladder, turned on his garden hose, and proceeded up the ladder to spray water on his roof. Eventually, the fire department arrived and put out the fire. It wasn't until latter that evening that G.H. again became aware of his back pain. Even then the pain did not seem as severe because he was now preoccupied with his harrowing experience and thinking about what needed to be done to cope with the damage.

Emergency situations such as this can override even intense pain signals. Although this example has little practical utility in the self-management of chronic pain, it does shed light on the basic nature of attention.

EXPLAINING HOW ATTENTIONAL PROCESSES WORK

It is often useful to provide patients with a basic rationale regarding how attention and perception work (McCaul & Malott, 1984). We begin by pointing out the selective nature of perception. While awake, the mind is potentially able to perceive a considerable array of information (input) from within the body and the external environment. It is not possible for the mind to be simultaneously aware of all available input, otherwise it would become overwhelmed. As a result, the mind works in a selective manner, attending to some information and filtering out other input. It is analogous to a spotlight in a large arena illuminating some objects and leaving others in darkness. At some point it may be instructive to stop speaking and ask patients to pay close attention to each sound in the room. Usually, participants suddenly become aware of subtle sounds: the hum of an air conditioner or heating system, the ticking of a clock, the sound of others breathing, faint noises from outside the room, etc. It is pointed out that although those background sounds existed all along, they were not attended to and perceived while the instructor was talking. The mind tends to focus on incoming information that is more important, relevant, or novel, whereas other types of input are ignored or fade away. There is no question that acute pain sensations are important and relevant information, since they represent a threat to the integrity of the body. Chronic pain, on the other hand, usually fails to serve any useful informational function.

One important distinction regarding attentional focus is between internal sensory input and external environmental input. Attention can oscillate between these sources of input. A simple experiment can illustrate this. Patients are given the following instructions:

Just close your eyes and become very aware of some part of your body that you associate with pain. Notice carefully the sensations coming from that part right now. What do those sensations feel like? . . . (pause) . . . *And now open your eyes and begin looking very closely at* . . . (name some object in the room). *Look at it closely, noticing its size, shape, and color. Try to focus all of your attention, all of your awareness right now on this* . . . (object). *Just keep studying it as though you were seeing it for the first time* . . .

Patients are then asked at what point they were most aware of pain. Most will admit this occurred during the first part of the experiment. Awareness of an external object results in less awareness of internal bodily stimuli.

The extent to which one attends to internal versus external stimuli depends in part on the degree of competition among available cues (Pennebaker, 1982). The probability that an internal or external stimulus will be attended to depends on the number and nature of competing cues. Pain stimuli by nature are powerful cues that compete with perception of external stimuli. Thus, people in pain are often less aware of their external environment. The process of perception, however, involves more than passively registering stimulus information. It is also an active process that can be influenced by emotional factors. Pain, being a highly aversive stimulus, elicits emotional arousal. This arousal is also enhanced when the individual feels unable to control and terminate the pain sensations. Consequently, attention is directed not only to the sensory aspects of pain but also to the negative emotional arousal (suffering component). This emotional arousal can have two negative consequences. First, it results in a narrowing of attention. There is an increased focus on somatic sensations and emotional distress. Second, the arousal can have adverse physiological consequences. As a result of increased muscle tension and autonomic arousal, the original pain sensations are amplified, and additional unpleasant sensations can arise (e.g., tension headache). In other words, vicious cycles are created resulting in ever increasing somatic preoccupation, emotional distress, and self-preoccupation.

The typical ways in which these patients cope behaviorally with pain also tend to reduce the number of potential competing external cues. Social withdrawal and inactivity facilitate increased attention to internal stimuli. Narcotic use not only blunts awareness of internal sensations but also interferes with perception of external stimuli. It is thus repeatedly stressed how all these vicious cycles contribute to chronic pain and suffering.

In addition to a lack of competing cues and increased emotional arousal, attention to pain sensations can be facilitated through the presence of particular environmental cues. For example, inquiries from well-meaning family members and friends regarding the patient's health or pain level can increase pain awareness. Simple questions such as "How are you feeling today?" or "Are you having much pain right now?" serve as cues to focus attention on somatic sensations. Visits to physicians, medical clinics, and hospitals can also provide multiple cues to direct attention to pain and other unpleasant sensations. It has been our impression that when some patients visit a pain clinic or are admitted to a hospital-based pain program they immediately become more attentive to their pain because of all these cues.

ATTENTION DIVERSION AND
SELF-MANAGEMENT TRAINING

An important issue in pain programs is the relative degree of emphasis placed on distraction as a pain management strategy. It is our impression that it is often given too little attention. Perhaps this is because the very idea of attention diversion is so simple and within the realm of common sense. Unfortunately, some professionals have used it to give patients superficial and pat advice when asked what can be done, apart from drugs, to cope with chronic pain. For example, it is tempting to tell patients, "Just keep busy and try not to think about your pain," or "Turn your mind to something else." This advice, probably like most advice, is much easier to deliver than it is to implement. Attention diversion also lacks the "glamor" of many other common pain-management approaches such as hypnosis, biofeedback, acupuncture, electrical nerve stimulation, drugs, injections, etc. Unlike distraction, the administration of these techniques requires special training or professional certification. Nevertheless, the use of attention diversion should be given the emphasis it deserves as one of the most valuable and practical approaches to pain management.

Especially important is the recognition that diversion of attention from pain will be enhanced by increasing the availability of distracting environmental stimuli. Consequently, a major focus of self-management training should be to encourage and assist patients to engage in a variety of distracting activities. This particularly applies to those who have become socially withdrawn, inactive, sedentary, or even bedridden as part of their chronic-pain syndrome. Participation in a variety of interesting and rewarding activities can significantly counteract the vicious cycle associated with pain preoccupation and misery.

In addition to distracting activity, patients are taught and encouraged to generate their own cognitive distractions in the absence of external stimulus input. Relaxation procedures, meditative approaches, and imagery techniques can be used for such purposes. At the same time, the focus on cognitive distractions should be kept in perspective. It is noteworthy that most discussions of distraction in the professional literature refer more to cognitive strategies (e.g., attention to breathing, use of visual focus points, listening to music or sounds, various types of mental activity, and imagery) than to maintenance of a healthy and balanced activity level. For example, in McCaffery's (1979) excellent discussion of distraction, she devotes most of her attention to cognitive strategies that can be used to relieve pain for brief periods of time. Although special cognitive distraction exercises are of value, we believe that engaging in a variety of stimulating daily activities has much greater potential benefit for those with chronic, continuous pain. Activities which require focused attention for their execution can have the effect of automatically distracting attention away from pain for much greater periods of time than special cognitive distraction techniques.

DISTRACTING ACTIVITIES

Distracting activities fall into three general areas: work, recreation, and social activities (Sternbach, 1987). Work includes not only paid employment, but also a variety of other work-like activities. Recreational activities can include any number of hobbies and leisure time pursuits that the person finds relaxing, stimulating, or enjoyable. Interaction with other people, provided the focus of attention is not on pain and related problems, can also be a useful distraction along with providing many other benefits.

Work

Vocational or other work-like activities can serve as a major source of distraction as well as provide many other tangible and intangible rewards for those with chronic pain. For the majority of adults, work activities consume a large portion of waking hours. Paid employment, self-employment, household chores, child care, and volunteer work not only occupy considerable time and attention but can also contribute to life satisfaction and self-worth. Many individuals derive considerable meaning, purpose, and a sense of productivity from these activities. Thus, part of the total evaluation of those who have entered a chronic-pain program should include assessment of the patient's vocational history, status, goals, and potential.

Those who are currently employed or have significant work-like responsibilities, such as housework and child care, usually require assistance in more effectively managing the physical and stressful demands of these responsibilities. It is especially important that these individuals learn more effective means of managing work-related stress as well as learning how better to pace themselves and modulate specific physical tasks. These issues are discussed in Chapters 4 and 7. The concern here is with those who have few work-like responsibilities, are unemployed, or are on temporary work disability. These individuals must be encouraged and assisted to develop specific goals in the above mentioned areas. Some are able to return to their previous occupations or places of employment. Others may need to be retrained for another type of work. In such cases, referral to a vocational rehabilitation specialist or evaluation center is recommended. These specialists can provide a more thorough and comprehensive assessment of the patient's vocational interests, aptitudes, and skills. In collaboration with the patient, specialists can then discuss employment alternatives, training requirements of specific occupations, public and private vocational training and assistance resources, and employment opportunities.

Irrespective of the availability of vocational rehabilitation specialists, a primary goal of a pain management staff is to stimulate the patient's desire to return to work. We also attempt to instill confidence that patients can successfully meet work demands without significantly increasing their pain. Even though it is assumed that disability compensation serves as a powerful counterincentive to return to gainful employment, the focus should be on how the individual pain patient appraises his or her own prospects of returning to work. Few will actually state a preference for receiving disability compensation over earned income. Rather patients may say, "I really don't like the idea of living on disability, and I really would rather be working, but I have no choice." One common objection to employment is patients' belief that they are unable to meet the physical demands of their preferred work without significantly injuring themselves or exacerbating their pain condition. The major self-management principles used to counter this objection were discussed in the previous chapter. Patients must establish and maintain a physical reconditioning program, work toward accurately determining their true physical limitations, learn how to pace physical activities effectively, and establish reasonable goals regarding the types of work activities or employment alternatives that are possible.

Another common objection among patients is the belief that no employer would be willing to hire them because of their medical history. It should be acknowledged that some employers may be reluctant to hire an individual with chronic back pain or other disabilities because of concerns relating to increased insurance and liability risk. However, it is also the case that many employers are willing to hire such individuals providing they are qualified and able to do the job. Consequently, many individuals with a history of chronic pain or even severe physical disabilities are gainfully employed. It is often helpful to refer to specific examples of individuals with chronic-pain conditions who are gainfully employed.

Some potential reasons for a reluctance to return to work are less likely to be openly admitted or even consciously recognized. For some, a chronic-pain condition can serve as a convenient "self-handicapping" strategy to excuse them for failing to meet their own vocational aspirations or living up to the expectations of significant others. They can then say to themselves or others, "I could have been a success at . . . if it hadn't been for my pain condition (injury, disease, surgery, etc.)." This face-saving device can enable patients to avoid facing insecurities regarding their skills, failure to meet their achievement goals, or unrealistic self-expectations and standards of success. Some also use pain as an excuse to avoid returning to a previously held job that was considered boring and unrewarding or overly stressful and demanding. These underlying reasons for failing to make honest efforts to return to work can be discovered and tactfully pointed out to patients during the course of individual counseling or in group therapy.

At the same time, it is recognized that return to gainful employment may be an inappropriate goal for some pain patients. Those who are beyond retirement age constitute the most obvious example. Nevertheless, it is important that we not automatically assume that everyone who is beyond a certain age is disinterested or inappropriate for vocational counseling or retraining. The same point can be made for those with significant physical limitations. Although such limitations can interfere with many types of work, it is possible for some with even severe physical disabilities to become employed after being trained to use various types of adaptive equipment. Other factors that contribute to poor potential for return to work include unstable employment history before onset of the pain problem, limited work skills, low aptitude for vocational training, and lengthy periods of unemployment prior to or following the disability. Irrespective of the reason, those who are either inappropriate candidates for vocational retraining or unlikely to return to work can be encouraged to find alternative work-like activities that will not only occupy their attention but will also enable them to feel useful and productive. As noted earlier, many of our pain program graduates have discovered rewards in volunteer activities including work with the physically ill, disabled, elderly, economically disadvantaged, youth groups, etc.

Recreation

In addition to work and work-like activities, hobbies and leisure-time pursuits can serve as significant distractions from chronic pain. Many chronic-pain patients do report engaging in a particular hobby as a way of distracting their attention from pain. Although such adaptive behavior should be encouraged, it may appear that some patients spend an excessive amount of time at one particular passive activity such as reading. These individuals can be encouraged to develop additional leisure activities to add more variety to their lives. Unfortunately, many have discontinued their hobbies and recreational activities after developing a chronic-pain problem. Some will admit that they just do not feel like pursuing activities that they previously had found enjoyable. This is a likely symptom of depression. More frequently, patients state that they are incapable of engaging in specific activities because of their pain condition. In such cases, it is necessary to ascertain whether pain is serving as an excuse to mask their depression.

On the other hand, some leisure-time activities may need to be abandoned because they are too physically demanding and exceed the patient's limits. This is particularly relevant for those who had engaged in vigorous sporting activities prior to their pain condition. These individuals should be encouraged to find alternative, less physically demanding activities. This may entail developing new hobbies and leisure-time activities, or it may involve modifying previously enjoyed physically demanding activities. Examples of such modifications can be drawn from the reports of many pain patients. One individual who previously preferred backpacking in wilderness areas found he could still enjoy camping from his car. Another individual who had enjoyed stream fishing that involved considerable walking learned to enjoy fishing seated in a boat or on a pier. Some who had previously engaged in vigorous sporting events became coaches for little league groups. The process of making such modifications often requires confronting distorted, all-or-nothing thinking (e.g., "Either I do it the way I used to do it or I won't do it at all").

Finally, we make an effort to expose our patients to new activities that may evolve into hobbies or even vocational possibilities. Participants in our inpatient program are required to spend at least an hour a day engaging in some manual activity that is well within their limits. Facilities and instructors are available to assist them in working with wood or metal, photographing and developing pictures, gardening, lapidary and jewelry making, learning how to use a ham radio or CB radio, working with stained glass, etc. Many who previously had been very inactive and preoccupied with their pain discover that during the course of such activities they completely forget their pain.

Social Activity

The third major type of distracting activity is an especially important issue for those who have withdrawn from interacting with other people as part of their chronic-pain syndrome. Fortunately, participation in a group program can significantly counteract this tendency. Prior to entering such a program, the patient may have felt alone or thought that no one could understand his or her situation. Since many do report considerable benefit from interacting with others who have chronic pain, the development of pain support groups should be encouraged. Such groups can either be professionally led or self-led. We offer a weekly support group for pain patients who have completed our intensive inpatient program as well as for those who do not desire or require such a program. As group leaders, we attempt to present, review, and initiate discussion of pain self-management principles and techniques. Additionally, those who attend this group report considerable benefit from the information, encouragement, and support provided by other group members. Many also state that the group helps them maintain a better perspective on their problems. Once each month this group is led by a nonprofessionally trained person who is a successful graduate of our pain program and now employed as our administrative coordinator. These sessions are especially useful for those who have difficulty accepting guidance from professionals who have not themselves experienced chronic pain. Peer-led self-help groups can serve as a significant source of social support and encouragement.

Social activities must extend beyond interaction with others with chronic pain. As a form of distraction, pain support groups are of limited value. Interaction with family and friends can provide much more extensive distraction from pain, providing the focus of conversation is not on pain or related problems. Patients are discouraged from discussing and complaining about pain to family and friends. Most are willing to admit that such discussions are of little value and only serve to keep attention focused on pain. Additionally, family and friends often tire of listening to recurrent pain complaints, since there is relatively little they can do to help the person in pain feel more comfortable. However, as mentioned earlier, inquiries from some well-meaning family members and friends often occur that direct attention toward the patient's pain. Patients should be advised to take the responsibility to let these individuals know that such inquiries are not helpful and inform them how they can be more helpful. For example, when a question is raised regarding how the person with pain is feeling on a particular day, the well-meaning friend can be told, "I do appreciate your concern; however, you can be much more helpful to me if you can help me get my mind off my pain by talking about something other than my pain or how I'm feeling. In fact, I really enjoy it when we talk about. . . . "

Ideally, family members should be included in the patient's pain self-management training program. After the role of attention and distraction are explained, family members are advised either to ignore pain complaints and other pain behaviors or make efforts to respond to such behavior by directing conversation to something else. Family can also initiate and encourage the patient to participate in social activities. Patients and families are encouraged to become involved in various social organizations or join groups that are formed around special areas of interest. Family gatherings, church activities, community and neighborhood activities, sporting events, and work-related social events not only distract from pain but also provide other valuable benefits to the person in pain.

Activity Balance

Additionally, we recommend finding a healthy balance in the proportion of time allotted to each of these three areas. Although "healthy balance" must be individually determined, one general guideline is the ratio of "shoulds" to "wants" (Marlatt, 1985). Shoulds refer to activities perceived as external demands or requirements. They are done out of a sense of duty, responsibility, obligation, or necessity. Wants, on the other hand, are perceived primarily as enjoyable, pleasurable, and self-fulfilling. A preponderance of shoulds over wants is more likely to be associated with increased stress and a perception of self-deprivation. An excess of wants over shoulds can mean that one is failing to meet responsibilities and is not accomplishing things that need to be accomplished. It is recommended that pain patients closely examine their own patterns of daily activities to determine the degree of lifestyle balance. When imbalance is found, specific activity goals can be established to achieve greater balance.

Another important point regarding attention–diversion activities is that they are not necessarily healthy or beneficial to the person in the long run. Activities and events that are stressful and demanding can temporarily divert attention away from pain, but the adverse consequences of increased tension and pain may be experienced later. Even many nondemanding, enjoyable activities can elicit increased pain if persisted in too long. For example, one of our patients came to a group session complaining of increased neck pain. When questioned regarding what may have triggered the pain increase, the patient replied that he could not think of anything. One of the other group participants then noted that he had observed the patient bending over a "paint by numbers" project for several hours without a break the previous evening. The patient quickly replied that he wanted to finish the project and that he had been doing just what we had recommended by spending time in a distracting activity. Unfortunately, the fact that he had kept his neck in a flexed position for such a long time triggered the pain increase. As emphasized in the previous chapter, self-management of physical activities, including distracting activities, requires attention to posture, body mechanics, and pacing techniques.

COGNITIVE DISTRACTIONS

Although a good balance of work, recreation, and social activities is of greatest value in distracting attention away from pain, it is important to remember that constant activity is neither ideal nor possible. For example, many persons with chronic pain report success in keeping their attention diverted from pain during much of the day. Difficult times occur when they are no longer as active, such as in the evening or especially after they retire to bed. Many believe that the primary reason they experience greater pain at such times is that their bodies are actually hurting more. When discussing this problem with patients, one can suggest that increased pain awareness may also result from a lack of distracting activities rather than an increase in pain signals. At night, when the lights are off and after everyone else is asleep, awareness of pain can be especially high. This is one reason why many chronic-pain patients suffer from sleep disturbance.

Consequently, it is desirable for patients to learn how to distract themselves more effectively during periods of relative inactivity or when they are exposed to minimal environmental stimulation. When we are engaged in tasks that require concentration, attention is more or less automatically drawn to the task at hand. The same can be said when we are exposed to novel stimuli or are confronting environmental events that seem to demand our attention. During such times, we experience attention as the phenonemon of being "pulled" toward the relevant stimulus. Cognitive distraction techniques, on the other hand, are employed in a more conscious and deliberate manner. The person in pain must make a voluntary effort to redirect attention to some other nonpain object. This other object may be a physical object in the environment, alternative physical sensations, or mental phenomena (i.e., distracting thoughts and images).

Cognitive distraction techniques are first introduced in the context of relaxation-training exercises. These exercises are performed in a quiet environment, usually with the eyes closed to facilitate the withdrawal of attention from external stimuli. Participants are initially asked to direct their attention to the verbal instructions of the teacher. Eventually, they are required to generate their own instructions for attentional focus. Attention may be directed to the process of breathing, various muscle groups within the body, repetitive relaxing phrases, or relaxing images. Guidelines for relaxation training along with examples of specific relaxation exercises are discussed more fully in Chapter 7.

Attention can also be deliberately directed to environmental stimuli. Techniques referred to as "external focus" procedures involve attending to and concentrating on either visual or auditory stimuli. A specific visual stimulus may be selected, and the patient asked to look closely and carefully at it. This stimulus may be as simple as a spot on a wall or ceiling, or it may be a stationary object (e.g., a flower, candle flame, statue, wood carving, vase, painting, etc.). In some cases, patients are asked to fixate their gaze on the chosen object without excessively straining the eyes, whereas in other cases, eye strain is purposefully induced as a prelude to eye closure. The particular object chosen is not important providing it is either monotonous and uninteresting (e.g., a small hole in a ceiling tile), or interesting in such a way that it does not evoke an associative train of thought resulting in tension, anxiety, or other unpleasant emotions. For example, one of our patients, while focusing on a toy automobile, was reminded of the auto accident that had caused his painful injury. Obviously, this was an inappropriate visual target for this particular patient. Nevertheless, patients using this technique can choose almost any number of visual objects depending on the environment they are in. Sounds can also be used as targets of attention. Many patients enjoy listening to music as a distraction from pain. Nature sounds can be especially relaxing such as the sound of rain, ocean waves, birds chirping, etc. In fact, we have a tape library of recorded nature sounds that we make available to our patients. Other monotonous sounds and background noises can be used as foci of attention. Irrespective of the audio stimuli chosen, the patient is instructed to concentrate and listen very closely to the sounds. Sounds can either simply be listened to as such or can be incorporated into distracting mental imagery.

Patients are also instructed to practice utilizing internally generated cognitive stimuli to distract attention away from pain. These thoughts and images may or may not be associated with relaxation. In fact, exciting thoughts can serve as good distractors. To demonstrate this, we ask patients to close their eyes and imagine having just won the lottery and then go through the process of deciding how they would spend their money. Although almost any train of thought or sequence of images can potentially distract attention away from pain, we recommend using cognitions that have a neutral or positive affective valence. Cognitions that are associated with negative emotional arousal, such as fear and anger, may successfully divert away from pain; however, the longer-term consequences may be increased tension and pain. For example, a person may become temporarily distracted while recalling a bitter feud with a former supervisor or imagining what might happen in the event of a major earthquake. However, the patient may then be left with feelings of anger or fear that might trigger additional memories of arguments and conflicts or anticipatory thoughts of other potential misfortunes.

More mundane or emotionally neutral thoughts can serve as attention diversions. Planning the next day's activities, preparing a shopping list, or preparing a recipe are good examples. A related technique that we have utilized is focused awareness on routine, everyday activities. Here we refer to recurring activities that have been performed so often that they are done in a more or less automatic manner and require very little attention. Examples include personal hygiene activities (e.g., taking a shower, shaving, combing or brushing hair, cleaning teeth), dressing and undressing, eating, driving a car to familiar places, etc. During the course of such activities, it is common for attention to drift and wander to many other things. The focused-attention exercise requires the person to concentrate and fully attend to the activity, especially its sensory aspects. For example, while taking a shower, the person might closely attend to the sensations of water striking various parts of the body, the temperature and force of the water, the feel of a soap bar in the hand, the process of drying after completing the shower, etc. When eating, the person might attend to the sight and smell of the food and carefully savor each bite or sip of a beverage. During some routine activities such as driving or walking along a familiar route, the person could try to look more closely at specific or novel features of the environment. One can start this exercise by having patients chose one particular activity for focused awareness and mentally practice doing it as a miniexperiment (i.e., "try it and just see what you notice"). The exercise can then be expanded to include other routine activities.

To give this assignment more credibility, it can be suggested that this simple exercise can help the person improve his or her basic ability to utilize distraction and gain greater control over the mind. It can also be noted that variations of this procedure are found in some non-Western meditative traditions. In contrast to concentrative forms of meditation in which awareness is restricted to one particular object, "opening-up" or mindfulness meditation involves being responsive to all stimuli that are immediately present in the internal and external environment (Shapiro, 1980). Although not designed as a pain distraction strategy, this practice can enable one to be more attentive, fully absorbed, and involved in whatever one is doing, whether or not the task actually requires a lot of concentration. Greater awareness of and involvement in the surrounding natural and social environments as opposed to self-absorption also contribute to a reduction in the subjective experience of pain.

For those who are familiar with various forms of meditation, it may be noted that "opening-up" or mindfulness forms of meditation would actually include full awareness of pain when such pain is part of a person's immediate internal environment. Close attention to pain sensations is another cognitive technique that has been recommended as a self-management strategy (Turk et al., 1983). When using this technique, patients are instructed to analyze the sensations in a somewhat detached, objective, "scientific" manner. The goal is simply to be aware of pain sensations without the negative emotional and cognitive concomitants. Specific pain sensations are simply noted as such without an attempt to resist them or mentally to elaborate on their meaning and implications. Although pain patients generally prefer distraction techniques, this strategy may be more effective when pain is at higher levels of intensity (McCaul & Malott, 1984). Invoking the old adage, "if you can't beat 'em, join 'em," we suggest that detached, nonemotional attention to pain sensations is one of many strategies that patients can try on a purely experimental basis when distraction proves difficult.

During self-management training, it is useful to have patients practice generating various types of specific distracting thoughts and images. A few examples that can be done in a group setting include the following:

1. Recall a happy event from your childhood.
2. Imagine that you and your loved ones are given an all-expenses-paid, 3-week vacation to anywhere in the world.
3. Imagine how you would design the house of your choice.
4. See if you can recall the words to a favorite poem or song.

Additional examples may be tailored to the interests and concerns of specific patients. For example, those with a mechanical orientation may wish to imagine designing, constructing, or repairing some object of interest. Parents with young children may imagine their offspring growing up and becoming successful, famous, etc. Older individuals can be encouraged to reminisce. Unmarried and unattached people can imagine meeting an interesting and desirable partner.

Occasionally we encounter individuals who feel uncomfortable with the idea of engaging in fantasy. Some have been frequently punished for this practice in the past (e.g., "stop daydreaming and pay attention") and have come to consider it wrong or vaguely sinful to indulge in such activities. We try to remind these individuals that imagery is a normal and natural activity and that it can be a very helpful, therapeutic means of controlling pain providing it is not done excessively (e.g., to avoid responsibilities) or at inappropriate times (e.g., while doing a task that requires concentration). If one feels uncomfortable with fantasies of future success, fame, achievement, good fortune, etc., there are many other types of distracting mental activity that can be used. The important point is that distracting thoughts and images should have personal relevance, interest, and meaning in order to be most effective. The philosopher Immanuel Kant was reported to have focused on the name of "Cicero" with its multifarious associations as an effective remedy for the occurrence of pain at night (Turk, Meichenbaum, & Genest, 1983). These authors make the point that although Cicero's name may not have the same effect on people today, an effort should be made to help patients discover specific thoughts and images that are most interesting and enjoyable to them. This is in contrast to the common tendency for therapists to prescribe a set of canned, ready-made images.

Finally, patients should be reminded that in order to really learn and make effective use of cognitive distraction techniques it is necessary to have a mind that is clear and unclouded by drugs and other mind-dulling chemicals. These include all narcotics, many types of tranquilizers and sleep medications, alcohol, marijuana, cocaine, and other illicit drugs.

SUMMARY

The ability to redirect attention away from pain is one of the most valuable self-management methods for living with chronic pain. To support and enhance its value, patients are given a simple rationale drawing on basic knowledge regarding the psychology of attention and perception. Two forms of distraction are distinguished. First are various behavioral activities, most of which automatically require attention in order to be performed. These activities include vocational and other work-like activities, hobbies and recreational endeavors, and social activities. Patients are assisted and encouraged to develop a healthy balance of activity from each of these three overlapping life spheres, recognizing that their value extends far beyond their role as pain distractors. Depending on particular areas of deficit, chronic-pain patients are aided in developing specific and reasonable self-management goals. Second, patients are taught and encouraged to develop on their own a variety of internally generated cognitive distraction methods that can be used in the absence of behavioral activity or environmental stimulation. These can include meditation and imagery techniques, reminiscence, making future plans, simple environmental focus procedures, and a nearly endless variety of other cognitive techniques.

CHAPTER 6

Coping with Episodes
of Intense Pain

A common objection raised by patients who are receiving training in psychological approaches to pain control is that such methods do not work when pain is at a high level of intensity. For example, we may hear a statement such as, "Doctor, I know that the distraction and relaxation exercises you are teaching me help, but when my pain is at its peak, nothing works." Or the patient may say, "The other day I tried that relaxation exercise, but I was hurting so bad that I just could not concentrate so I ended up having to take a pain pill." Objections such as these tend to be raised especially by those who have been dependent on the use of narcotic analgesics, minor tranquilizers, or other central nervous system depressants. Sometimes it appears as though these individuals are expecting psychological methods to work in a similar manner to these substances. It takes relatively little effort and time to retrieve a pill from one's medicine cabinet, whereas it may seem much more difficult to employ a cognitive coping strategy. Thus, we have found it useful to devote special attention to how self-management applies to intense pain episodes.

First, it is important to define the meaning of intense pain episodes. We make it very clear that we are referring to episodic exacerbations of patients' chronic pain rather than to the onset of new, acute pain. We remind patients that their memory usually enables them to discriminate between familiar chronic-pain sensations and other types of pain sensations. Pain sensations that are not part of their chronic pain may be signaling a new injury or disease process. For most patients who report chronic continuous pain, such episodes are defined as periods in which pain intensity is at a peak. When numerical rating scales are used, the therapist can refer to the higher numbers on the scale. Using the six-point system originally described by Budzynski, Stoyva, Adler, and Mullaney

(1973) and later discussed by Turk et al. (1983), intense pain would be considered a 5 (intense, incapacitating, excruciating pain), or possibly a 4 (horrible pain in which one can still perform nondemanding tasks). Of course, there is considerable variability among patients regarding the qualitative and temporal description of these peaks. Some report relatively brief episodes (e.g., a few seconds) of intense pain that are described in such terms as sharp, shooting, and stabbing sensations or intense muscle spasms. Often these brief episodes occur in clusters. Others report longer periods of intense, continuous aching pain lasting several hours. Patients who present chronic, intermittent pain problems such as migraine headaches also vary in terms of how they regard their intense pain episodes. Some report that each time they have pain it is at peak intensity. Others report more variability in the intensity of their intermittent pain episodes. For example, they may distinguish between mild headaches and severe headaches.

Once it is clarified with each patient what is meant by intense pain episodes, they can be given an overall self-management perspective regarding this problem. This approach consists of two basic components: (1) prevention and (2) use of constructive coping strategies.

PREVENTION

Prevention is obviously the preferred approach. However, it is predicated on the belief that pain intensity is under some degree of control through the patient's own actions. Although most chronic-pain patients accept this idea, some regard their intense pain episodes as completely random, unpredictable, and totally outside of their control.

We begin a discussion of prevention by introducing the concept of pain triggers. Pain triggers are defined as any situation, event, or activity that tends to elicit intense pain. Although not all intense pain episodes have an identifiable trigger, in our experience most chronic-pain patients are able to identify at least some pain triggers.

The usual recommendation for identifying such triggers is to require the patient to monitor his or her pain intensity over a period of time in order to identify situational determinants or temporal patterns of intense pain. Although regular pain intensity ratings were originally recommended primarily in research contexts, caution should be exercised in using this procedure in strictly clinical settings. We are particularly concerned with the requirement to record pain intensity ratings on an hourly basis during all waking hours. In order to comply fully with this requirement, the patient must interrupt whatever he or she is doing or attending to at least once each hour and direct attention to the pain (i.e., "how much am I hurting right now?"). This is, of course, directly counter to what we are trying to teach patients.

Rather than using hourly pain ratings on a routine basis with all patients, we recommend that such ratings be used only if needed. Most patients are able to identify pain triggers and temporal patterns in their pain intensity without going through the laborious and potentially countertherapuetic process of filling out hourly pain-intensity rating cards. If such pain ratings are used routinely, they should be used for a limited period of time (e.g., 2 weeks prior to beginning a self-management training program). Pain monitoring may be more appropriate for those who present intermittent pain problems, such as headaches. In this case, they are not asked to rate pain on an hourly basis. Rather, they are required to record information regarding each headache episode including antecedent factors and coping responses.

One potential difficulty concerns the temporal relationship between situational triggers and the occurrence of intense pain. It is much easier to identify triggers when pain intensity increases concurrently with or shortly after the occurrence of the trigger. For some, however, there is a temporal delay between the triggering event and the pain. A person with chronic back pain may experience an exacerbation the day following an episode of heavy lifting. Some individuals experience migraine attacks after a period of stress has presumably ended (e.g., on weekends or during a vacation).

Uncontrollable versus Controllable Triggers

After the concept of pain triggers is introduced and some examples are identified, it is pointed out that triggers tend to fall into one of two categories: uncontrollable and potentially controllable. Uncontrollable triggers include those situations or events over which one has relatively little direct control. Unpredictable emergencies, unavoidable accidents, and certain weather conditions may be uncontrollable triggers for intense pain episodes. In such cases, prevention is not possible, and the patient is left with the second approach, which is to use a constructive pain-coping strategy.

The majority of pain triggers, on the other hand, are controllable, and thus they can be used as a basis for prevention. Most individuals are able to identify several controllable pain triggers. Some, on the other hand, have difficulty distinguishing between controllable and uncontrollable triggers. In this case, the patient may label a trigger as uncontrollable that is, in fact, potentially controllable. For example, a patient may refer to a particular physical chore that must be completed within a particular time frame or in a particular manner. The patient is in effect saying, "I had no choice in how I went about doing this physical task." Most often, other group members will point out the fallacy of uncontrollability. For those who have difficulty identifying any controllable triggers, we will sometimes ask, "If I could pay you enough money to increase your pain intensity significantly, what would you do?" Most patients respond to this challenge by mentioning several physical activities such as lifting a heavy object, sitting too long, walking too far, etc.

After some examples of controllable pain triggers are identified, it is pointed out that many of these fall into one of two general categories. First are those triggers pertaining to physical activities and exceeding physical limitations. Second are those triggers relating to tension, stress, and emotional arousal. Both are major self-management issues discussed in our program and covered at greater length in other chapters. Other controllable triggers, although much less common, are specific dietary behaviors, including alcohol and caffeine intake, and altered sleep patterns.

The fundamental point to be conveyed is that, to a certain degree, the experience of chronic pain is within the patient's own control. Episodes of intense pain do not always just happen to patients in a random and unpredictable manner. By exercising more effective management of daily physical activities and stressful life experiences, it is possible to exercise greater control over pain intensity. Thus, many chronic-pain exacerbations can be prevented by applying self-management principles.

Narcotic Dependence as a Trigger

Few patients are aware that the very method commonly used to treat intense pain can ultimately trigger intense pain episodes (Sternbach, 1987). The roots of this problem begin with the observation that most chronic-pain patients who use narcotics do so on a p.r.n. ("as needed") basis. This often means that patients wait until pain is especially intense before resorting to pills. Many will tell us, "I really hate having to take those drugs, but when my pain is at its peak, it is the only thing that helps." Unfortunately, during times of peak pain intensity, analgesics tend to be the least effective. This sets the stage for the consumption of ever-increasing quantities to achieve the desired level of pain relief. As higher doses or stronger types of narcotics are used, tolerance effects develop along with drug dependency. In time, failure to maintain constant narcotic intake elicits withdrawal reactions, and these withdrawal reactions act as physiological and psychological stressors that trigger increased pain (Gildenberg & DeVaul, 1985). In short, the repetitive cycle of pain relief and narcotic withdrawal perpetuates and intensifies the pain cycle.

These observations must be carefully explained, since they seem to run counter to the common belief that narcotic usage decreases pain rather than triggers intense pain. It should be emphasized that the common practice of p.r.n. analgesic use actually promotes drug dependence and withdrawal effects. Thus, as noted earlier, it is important to provide a thorough and convincing rationale for taking analgesics regularly according to fixed time intervals rather than as needed. In addition to using the time-interval approach to withdraw patients from narcotics, this method is recommended for patients who feel unable to cope with pain without analgesics. Fortunately, the time-interval method usually enables the patient to take less potent analgesics, since it tends to reduce the peaks and valleys of pain intensity. Ultimately, the real goal is complete elimination of all narcotics even though the process of withdrawal may temporarily increase pain perception.

Sensory Cues as Warning Triggers

Prevention of some intense pain episodes can also be accomplished without necessarily identifying an external pain trigger. Some patients are able to identify specific sensory warning signals that an intense pain episode is about to occur. For example, it is known that those who suffer from classic migraine episodes experience sensory changes approximately 15 to 30 minutes before onset of an actual attack. The most common of these are visual anomalies. Some are able to use these signals to abort an impending attack using a self-management strategy (e.g., a relaxation procedure, drinking coffee, physical activity). Some patients also experience more gradual increases in pain intensity. If this occurs in a predictable manner, it may be possible to use early pain signals as a cue to employ a preventive strategy. For example, rather than responding to these early signals by contracting the muscles, the patient may learn to relax these muscles thereby preventing a continued escalation in pain intensity.

CONSTRUCTIVE ALTERNATIVES
FOR COPING WITH PAIN

Since not all intense pain is preventable, it is necessary to consider the second component that involves use of constructive coping strategies while an intense pain episode is in effect. It is also recognized that consistently perfect prevention is unlikely in spite of good intentions. Furthermore, on some occasions a patient may choose to engage in a particular physical activity knowing full well that an intense pain episode will follow. In such cases, the patient may do a cost-benefit analysis before engaging in the activity and decide that the benefits of the activity outweigh the negative consequence of increased pain. Often, such activities are of a social nature. The patient is later able to use a constructive coping self-statement such as, "I had a great time, and even though I'm paying a price right now, it was worth it."

Constructive coping strategies are defined as actions that enable the person to self-manage time-limited episodes of intense pain without perpetuating the pain cycle. Rather than leaving the patient feeling overwhelmed and victimized by uncontrollable pain sensations, such actions represent positive steps that can enable him or her to maintain a perception of control. These strategies are also in contrast to destructive, self-defeating actions that are commonly used by patients seen in pain clinics. Narcotic use, visits to hospital emergency rooms, excessive alcohol consumption, social withdrawal, and prolonged inactivity are obvious examples of destructive pain-coping responses. Intense pain episodes also tend to elicit increased muscle tension, emotional distress, and a variety of negative images and self-statements. Examples of such statements include:

"I don't know if I can stand this pain much longer."
"Why can't those doctors do something for me?"
"This pain is driving me crazy."
"Why do I have to keep going through this suffering?"

Some report various negative images regarding immediate eliciting stimuli such as a picture of bone rubbing against an exposed, raw, hypersensitive nerve. Others dwell on memory images associated with the onset of their pain. For example, one may replay the events leading up to an injury. Another imagines angrily confronting a physician whom he holds responsible for the chronic-pain condition. Some patients imagine the dismal consequences of their bodies continuing to deteriorate. Unfortunately, it is during those times when pain is most severe that patients are most likely to engage in negative, destructive, and self-defeating coping efforts.

It is important to require each patient to go through a process of close self-examination to identify specific thoughts and actions that are most likely to occur during intense pain. Although some individuals can spontaneously report their accompanying cognitions, it is sometimes useful to ask them to imagine a recent severe pain episode or have them note their thoughts the next time such an episode occurs. It may be important to emphasize during this discussion that such actions and thoughts are very common and natural even though they are ultimately self-defeating and destructive. It is pointed out that, although some coping actions may reduce pain intensity in the short run, they ultimately tend to perpetuate the chronic-pain syndrome. Alcohol consumption, narcotic use, emergency room visits to receive an injection, and prolonged bed rest are typical examples. Other common coping reactions contribute to the pain cycle in a more immediate manner. By referring to the biopsychosocial model, health care professionals can remind patients how emotions, thoughts, actions, and physiological factors can interact and reciprocally influence each other in a negative way. For example, intense pain sensations associated with negative self-statements and distressing emotions are also accompanied by elevated muscle tension and autonomic arousal. These physiological reactions can interact with and exacerbate the original pain sensations, creating a vicious cycle. Another example is social withdrawal and bed rest, which both serve to remove the person from potential distractions and enable even greater self-absorption and preoccupation with the pain experience.

Developing Realistic Expectations

When discussing constructive coping strategies for intense pain, it is important to guide patients to realistic expectations. If expectations are too high, patients are likely to experience failure, which only serves to perpetuate the problem. For most people, complete eradication of the pain experience is an unrealistic goal. Although some are able eventually to become pain-free as a result of self-management training, it is unlikely that a constructive coping strategy employed in the midst of a particular intense pain episode will succeed in eliminating all pain. Most are willing to accept this, since even narcotic medication often fails to eliminate severe pain completely unless it is taken in doses high enough to disrupt conscious awareness significantly. Partial reduction in pain intensity is a more realistic goal and is acceptable to most patients.

To illustrate how partial reduction in pain intensity is possible, we use the vicious-cycle concept. Intense pain tends to elicit a number of negative emotional, cognitive, physiological, and behavioral reactions that, in turn, result in even greater pain and suffering. If one can replace these negative reactions with constructive coping alternatives, the vicious cycle is broken even though some pain remains. This reduced pain can then be viewed as tolerable and controllable as opposed to overwhelming and unbearable.

It is also useful at this point to remind patients of the gate-control model of pain (see Chapter 3). Although it is usually not possible to close the gate completely during severe pain, the gate can be closed at least to some degree. Some strategies presumably close the gate by altering patterns of peripheral stimulation to the spinal gate, whereas others close it by activating descending inhibitory mechanisms from the brain itself.

It is then suggested that patients have at least three general strategies that can be used to manage intense pain: (1) actions aimed at altering sensory stimulation, (2) distraction of attention, and (3) cognitive strategies directed at modifying the pain experience or reaction to pain. These general strategies are by no means mutually exclusive and may each be used in any one intense pain episode.

Altering Sensory Input

Attempts to alter sensory input directly can include many strategies patients have already been using prior to entering the pain program. In fact, it is often useful to have the group make a list of actions members have used on their own to cope with intense pain. Most of these actions tend to fall into one of four categories. First are attempts to alter sensory awareness through use of drugs or alcohol. Such attempts are seldom constructive. Second are those actions aimed at discontinuing the activity presumed to be exacerbating the pain in the first place. Lying down, standing up, changing positions, and retiring to a dark, quiet room are examples. The problem with these actions is that they merely disrupt ongoing goal-directed activities and are seldom seen as constructive, especially if prolonged. Third are attempts to divert attention away from the pain. Such attempts are often constructive and are referred to in the next section. Fourth are those actions that provide some form of counterstimulation. Examples include rubbing or massaging painful areas, applying wet or dry heat (e.g., hot shower, bath, jacuzzi, heating pad), applying ice packs, and doing gentle stretching exercises. We also include transcutaneous electrical stimulation (TENS) in this category even though it is not strictly a self-management procedure. Although some of these actions are viewed by professionals as classic pain behaviors (e.g., rubbing painful areas), we still label them as self-management actions. Other counterstimulation techniques, such as use of heat or cold and TENS, can be used in a constructive manner.

Distraction

Some individuals report attempts to distract attention away from intense pain. Such attempts are usually constructive and are obviously encouraged. As discussed in the preceding chapter, distraction can be a highly effective strategy for reducing pain awareness. At the same time, patients sometimes object to its value, claiming that distraction is not possible during episodes of intense pain. It is acknowledged that there is a marked tendency for intense pain to intrude on awareness, making distraction difficult to implement. Nevertheless, it is important for patients to discover the value of attention diversion even when pain is at a higher level of intensity. Patients are reminded of the relative interaction between pain awareness and distraction. Whereas it may not be difficult to divert attention from pain completely when pain is at a mild to moderate intensity level, it may be very difficult to do so when pain is severe. The relative interaction principle as discussed previously means that any degree of distraction results in less awareness of pain.

The choice of distracting activity during intense pain episodes is also an important consideration. The activity should not impose excessive physical demands that may exacerbate the pain. The degree of concentration required to engage in the activity should also be considered. If a great deal of concentration is required, the person may become frustrated since intense pain interferes with attention. On the other hand, if too little concentration is required, the activity may lose its distracting value unless the person makes an effort to concentrate. For example, it is possible to sit in front of a television set without really attending to the program. As a general principle, McCaffery (1979) suggests an inverted U-shaped relationship between pain intensity and the required complexity of the distraction. As pain increases, the complexity of the distraction should also increase. However, when pain is at a high intensity level, the distractor should be less complex. For relatively brief periods of intense pain, she recommends several distraction strategies including rhythmic breathing procedures, visual concentration on a point, singing and rhythmic tapping, auditory stimulation via earphone, and exposure to humorous books, recordings, etc.

Depending on the length of the intense pain episode, the person should have a variety of distracting activities available. In addition to limitations in concentration, a single activity, if engaged in too long, may put excessive strain on particular sensory and motor functions. The resulting mental and physical fatigue may exacerbate the ongoing pain. The specific choice of distracting activity will vary from person to person and situation to situation. Patients should be encouraged to be flexible and experiment with several distracting activities rather than relying on only one or two.

Cognitive Strategies to Alter the Pain Experience or Reactions to Pain

Rather than distracting attention away from intense pain, it may become necessary to acknowledge and work with the pain in a more constructive manner to limit its aversive effects. McCaul and Malott (1984) suggest that higher levels of pain stimulation are more effectively reduced by redefinition strategies that involve nonemotional attention to pain sensations. Since this approach is not as familiar to most chronic-pain patients, we usually devote more attention to it. A wide variety of redefinition strategies, self-instructional processes, and imagery techniques may be used.

Before discussing specific coping strategies, it is often useful to consider the patient's general orientation or attitude toward the experience of intense pain. Typically, intense pain is viewed as a very intrusive, distressing, frustrating, or even overwhelming event. The following three alternative constructive orientations (redefinitions) are suggested and discussed:

- Pain as a teacher or reminder
- Pain as an enemy
- Survival without resistance

Pain as a Teacher

Although chronic pain does not have the same useful warning function as acute pain, some find it useful to regard exacerbations of chronic pain as having potential warning value. When viewed in this way, intense pain sensations can be appraised as important messages from the body indicating the need for some type of corrective action. These messages usually pertain to either of two primary areas, emotional stress and overactivity.

> I.J. had a 10-year history of facial pain for which he had taken codeine for several years. During the course of self-management training, he became aware that he had a significant problem with anger. After being weaned from narcotics, he realized that the intensity of his facial pain directly reflected the degree of frustration and anger that he was experiencing at that time. Thus, he was able to utilize his pain as a cue or reminder that he needed to find a constructive means of handling his anger.

This approach serves to redefine pain exacerbations and give them a more positive meaning. The ultimate goal is to reduce emotional distress (suffering) as a direct response to intense pain episodes.

The pain-as-teacher orientation also has some limitations that should be noted. First, it is possible that some patients may respond to an episode of intense pain by becoming self-critical and self-punitive. For example, a patient who experiences intense pain as a result of exceeding his physical limitations may say to himself, "well I blew it again and overdid it. I just hate myself for not being able to do what I used to do; I guess there's no point in even trying to get any work done around this house." A more constructive alternative would be to view the pain as a message that the person must change the way in which he performs certain chores at home. Thus, it is essential that patients use pain feedback as a constructive learning experience rather than as a punishment. Another limitation is that increases in pain severity do not serve a useful informative function for many individuals. Since there is nothing to learn from the pain, alternative orientations must be used.

Pain as an Enemy

At first glance, this orientation might appear to be the one already maintained by almost all pain patients, although such is not the case. We view this strategy as a way of objectifying and distancing oneself from the immediate pain experience. This is in contrast to the usual tendency to identify fully with the pain experience (e.g., "I am in tremendous pain"). When presenting this as a constructive orientation, we point out that pain is a very tricky enemy that must be fought skillfully. It is further suggested that some of the major strategies employed by this enemy are to:

1. Get you upset and tense.
2. Make you feel depressed, helpless, and generally worthless as a human being.
3. Interfere with your life activities and keep you from enjoying anything.
4. Disrupt your social relationships, make you feel isolated, and create dissention within your family.
5. Turn you into a drug addict or alcoholic.

Unfortunately, the more successful pain is in accomplishing these objectives, the more powerful and controlling it becomes. For example, the common tendency to defend against intense pain with increased muscle tension and emotional distress is like fighting a fire with gasoline. Consequently, one must learn how to become a "skillful warrior" making use of all available self-management "weapons." In this regard, it may be useful to inform patients of some general principles utilized in many of the martial arts. Rather than attacking opponents in a blind, head-on manner, the skillful combatant stays loose and relaxed while being alert to the enemy's movements. When the enemy attacks, the combatant may try to redirect the blow so that it does the least damage. An attempt is made to conserve and utilize energy in an efficient manner. Excessive anger and muscle tension are seen as wasteful uses of energy. Controlled, relaxed breathing is very important. With continued practice, the various techniques become more automatic and flexible in their application.

The pain-as-enemy orientation can also be useful in channeling anger in a more constructive fashion. Rather than suppressing anger, turning it inward, or directing it against family, friends, health care providers, or the disability compensation system, the patient is encouraged to direct anger at the enemy to keep it from accomplishing its agenda. Anger then can be used as a motivating force to enable one to develop more constructive outlets and to achieve goals.

One potential problem in using the pain-as-enemy orientation is that it may elicit thoughts of finding ways to defeat and destroy the enemy. Since total eradication of pain may not be possible, the patient may have to be reminded that, even though the enemy is too strong to be completely destroyed at the present time, it is still possible to keep the enemy from destroying or getting the best of him or her. In other words, the primary goal is to keep the pain enemy from getting the upper hand.

Surviving Intense Pain while Minimizing Resistance

Another general orientation toward pain that acknowledges its strength without allowing it to become overwhelming is the concept of least resistance. This approach involves two key principles. The first principle is to avoid directly fighting and resisting intense pain sensations, since this only serves to create additional tension and frustration, thereby fueling a vicious cycle. This can be illustrated through various concrete metaphors. One metaphor that we find useful, since we live in Southern California, is that of the surfer or ocean swimmer. Intense pain sensations are analogous to huge ocean waves. It is impossible to stop these waves, and if one attempts to meet them with direct resistance, the person will be knocked over. Thus, the goal is to become like a surfer who knows how to ride the wave. As the wave peaks and descends, the person learns to flow with the wave rather than fighting it. Another metaphor for intense pain is a storm. Storms cannot be stopped; rather, they must be weathered. Realistic goals are to seek shelter, prevent damage, survive, and stay as comfortable as possible while the storm is raging.

The second key principle is to recognize that intense pain is a time-limited phenomenon. In the midst of intense pain, it is common for a person to lose this temporal perspective. Although the duration is variable, intense pain should be viewed as an episodic occurrence with a beginning and an end. It may begin and end abruptly or gradually. In a similar manner, storms can also be seen as time-limited. They eventually end, and when they do, one can experience a tremendous sense of relief. If shelter is not possible, one can become like a tree that bends with the wind but does not break. Each of these metaphors can be used to generate specific imagery that may be used during the intense pain episode. Again, the main idea to convey here is to flow with or relax through intense pain episodes without directly fighting or resisting until the intensity subsides.

Self-Instructional Processes

When confronting an intense pain episode, patients are encouraged to talk to themselves in a constructive manner. A basis for this approach is found in Meichenbaum's (1977) stress inoculation training procedure that was adapted for chronic-pain patients by Turk et al. (1983). This process can be presented as a way of using "positive self-suggestions" enabling patients to "psych themselves through times of intense pain." The specific content of this self-talk depends somewhat on the general orientation adopted by the patient. For example, if the pain-as-teacher orientation is used, appropriate self-statements may include:

"What is this pain telling me?"

"It looks like this pain is telling me that I overdid it yesterday when I cleaned the kitchen and bathroom floors. Next time I need to remember to take rest breaks rather than trying to do it all at once."

"I guess this pain is my body's way of letting me know that I'm letting myself get too tense over this situation."

"I'd better go do some time-out relaxation."

Examples of self-statements that may follow a pain-as-enemy orientation include:

"I'm going to just stay cool and not let this pain get the best of me."

"This pain is up to its old tricks again trying to get me down and discouraged, only I'm not going to let it."

"Keep hanging in there; the pain is making its attack now, but soon it will run out of steam, and I'll be the winner."

Sometimes self-statements may be expressed as messages to the pain itself. Such statements may be accompanied by anger and defiance. Some examples include:

"Go ahead and try to beat me down. I'll show you who's boss."

"There you go trying to trick me into taking drugs again. Well it's not going to work because I can handle you with my self-management techniques."

"Ok, so you're giving me a real rough time now. I'll fix you by just ignoring you and focusing my attention on this beautiful painting here."

When an attempt is made to survive without resisting, appropriate self-statements may include:

"Stay calm, don't get excited, just keep breathing slowly and
deeply."

"You're starting to get tense; just relax those muscles and flow with
it."

"I know it hurts right now, but I've been through this before. I know
I can handle it because it's not going to last."

The above self-statements are offered as examples. Rather than feed
patients with specific canned words or phrases, it is important to encourage and assist them to develop self-talk using their own words.

Pain Transformation Imagery

Mental imagery is another general coping strategy that can be used to
manage intense pain episodes. Although mental imagery was discussed in
Chapter 5 as a distraction technique, the focus here is on specific imaginal
procedures that acknowledge the existence of the pain. These procedures
use imagery to transform the meaning of the pain.

As with all self-management techniques, an attempt should be made
to give patients a reasonable and convincing rationale for the use of pain
transformation imagery. An example of such a rationale is as follows:

*Since all pain is ultimately received in the brain, mental imagery can be a powerful
tool to change the way in which the mind or brain interprets and responds to pain.
As we know, the mind does not respond very well to direct commands to reduce or
eliminate pain. For example, it usually doesn't work to say to oneself, "pain go
away" or "I'm not having pain." On the other hand, the mind does seem to be very
responsive to the use of imagination. If one can imagine something intensely and
really experience it, the mind responds as though the situation is actually true.
Mental imagery is a way to influence the mind into lessening the severity of pain or
reducing its negative impact.*

Sometimes it is useful to refer to the popular notion that we use only a
small part of our brain. Thus, it is possible through use of mental imagery
to make greater use of or expand the powers of the mind. Although
professionals who consider themselves strict empiricists may object to the
use of such language, we believe it is entirely justified when it helps to
mobilize patients' positive expectations.

Several types of pain transformation imagery are available. In a
classification system of cognitive coping strategies for pain developed by
Fernandez (1986), three types of transformation imagery are suggested:
contextual transformation, stimulus transformation, and response
transformation. Contextual transformation involves use of imagery to
change the setting or context within which the pain occurs. In other

words, although the pain is acknowledged, the situation is modified in a way that alters the reason for the pain's existence, thus giving it a more positive meaning. For example, a person with hip and leg pain may imagine that he was hurt during the course of a football game but is continuing to play, and perhaps even scoring the winning touchdown, in spite of the pain. Most of the examples cited in the literature involve similar heroic fantasies. The classic example, used originally by Knox (1973) in a laboratory pain study, is that of a spy who is shot in the arm and attempting to escape from enemy agents down a tortuous mountain road.

Stimulus transformation involves use of imagery to modify the immediate cause of the pain sensations. Some patients spontaneously report vivid images regarding pain-eliciting stimuli. Additionally, it may be useful to ask a patient to draw a picture of the pain. Examples of pain-eliciting images include nerves being stretched or tied up in knots, ice picks, daggers or bolts of electricity penetrating the body, vises clamping down or squeezing various body parts, hammers pounding on the skull, burning flames, etc. Once these spontaneous pain-eliciting images are identified, an effort can be made to modify them in a way that reduces pain intensity or changes the stimulus quality of the pain. Knots can be untied or at least loosened, ice picks can be removed, electricity can be grounded, vises can be loosened, hammer blows can be softened, fires extinguished, etc.

Response-transformation imagery involves relabeling, dissociating, or transforming the sensations arising from pain without reference to the concept of pain. For example, aching sensations can be relabeled as tingling, or specific aspects of the pain such as burning sensations can be focused on and dissociated from the totality of the pain experience. Some are able to use imagery to transform pain into numbness. For example, one might imagine a painful area as comprised of a block of wood that is insensitive to all feeling. We have also successfully used an old hypnotic technique, glove anesthesia, as a type of transformation imagery. In this technique, imagery is used to create a sense of numbness in one of the hands. For example, in one version described by Bresler (1979), the person imagines submerging his hand into a bucket containing a powerful anesthetic liquid that is easily absorbed through the pores of the skin. Once anesthesia is experienced, the patient can be taught to transfer it from the hand to a painful area of the body (e.g., placing the hand on a painful knee).

Another example of response-transformation imagery popular with many of our patients, involves imagining use of their own endorphins to elicit pain relief. Borrowing from a guided imagery procedure suggested by Olshan (1980), we have patients imagine the increased production of powerful pain-relieving chemicals in their brain and traveling directly to painful areas or to the spinal cord where they block the pain gate.

Specific types of pain-transformation imagery are almost limitless and depend largely on the therapist's and patient's imagination. During formal self-management training, we attempt to explain the general purpose of pain-transformation imagery, provide patients with concrete examples of such imagery, and then help them develop their own imagery. The most effective types of transformation imagery are those that relate to their ongoing natural pain images and are in accord with existing beliefs. For example, one patient was totally unable to use pain-projection imagery (i.e., projecting pain to an inanimate object) but responded very well to imagining mobilization of his endorphins. He stated afterwards that the idea of projecting his pain to an external object made absolutely no sense; however, the idea of mobilizing his endorphins made considerable sense, since he knew from prior reading that endorphins really existed.

Application of Pain-Coping Procedures

When discussing the use of various coping strategies for intense pain, it is useful to employ the "tools" metaphor. Each strategy represents a specific tool. In order to make good use of a tool, it is necessary to practice and become proficient in its use. Furthermore, a person who possesses only one or two tools is very limited in what can be accomplished. Ideally, one should be equipped with a variety of tools that can be used at different times and in different situations. Since the same tool does not work in every situation, it is necessary to be flexible and experimental. If a specific tool is not effective on a particular occasion, the person must guard against discouragement and simply try a different tool.

Unfortunately, while in the midst of intense pain, it is easy to forget the variety of tools that are potentially available. This is especially true in the earlier stages of self-management training before the use of these tools becomes habitual and automatic. At such times, patients are most likely to resort to earlier and often unhealthy habits such as taking narcotic analgesics. Thus, we require patients to develop their own list of constructive pain-coping tools. These lists are headed with the statement, "Things to do or think about when I am in intense pain." The list should be specific and include both cognitive and behavioral strategies. Only those strategies that are considered potentially helpful should be included. An example of one such a list can be seen in Table 6.1. The initial list can also be modified as one attains experience and attempts new coping strategies. To make use of the list, one must review it as one is experiencing an intense pain episode. Consequently, it should be posted in a visible location at home and carried in one's wallet or handbag.

TABLE 6.1.   Coping Strategies for Intense Pain Episodes: Things to Do
or Think about when Experiencing Intense Pain:

1. Stop and ask myself if I can identify the pain trigger or learn anything from this
   pain.
2. Begin slow, deep breathing and remind myself to keep calm; review my
   alternatives.
3. Identify some distracting activities, for example, conversation with my husband about anything other than pain, write a letter to a friend, do crossword
   puzzles, watch interesting TV program, bake cookies, prepare shopping list,
   go for a relaxing walk.
4. Take a long, hot shower.
5. Listen to one of my relaxation or self-hypnosis tapes.
6. Use positive self-reminders: the pain won't last; I can handle this on my own; I
   won't let it get the best of me; take it one step at a time; I've been through this
   before.
7. Use pain modification imagery: for example, imagine a block of ice resting on
   my back, see my endorphins working, transfer my pain to a block of wood.

Another useful training strategy, recommended by Turk et al.
(1973), is imaginal rehearsal of pain-coping techniques. Patients can be
asked to imagine undergoing an intense pain episode while employing
various constructive coping strategies. A debriefing process can also be
used with patients who have intense pain episodes as they go through the
pain program. Patients are asked to describe in detail the antecedents of
the episode along with the specific coping strategies used. They are then
asked to consider alternative actions that might have facilitated their
efforts to manage the pain.

Coping with Temptations to Use Drugs

Some patients who have been narcotic-dependent report much difficulty
coping with intense pain as they are being tapered off medication or
shortly after they have discontinued use of these drugs. It is during times
of intense pain that the desire is strongest to use mind-altering chemicals
to achieve relief. This dilemma is very similar to what is commonly faced
by cigarette smokers, alcoholics, and drug addicts after they have made a
commitment to abstain and have actually refrained from substance use for
a period of time. According to Marlatt and Gordon's (1985) relapse model,
control over substance use is threatened when former addicts encounter a
"high-risk situation." A high-risk situation is any situation that triggers
temptations to use the substance the subject has decided to refrain from.

Whether or not a lapse occurs depends heavily on whether the subject uses an appropriate coping strategy. Intense pain episodes are obviously significant high-risk situations for chronic-pain patients who have made a commitment to abstain from narcotics. This is particularly the case when these patients are at home and not surrounded by support from the program and when narcotics are readily available. It is very important that patients who are going through a pain-management program while being detoxified from narcotics anticipate this situation and develop preparatory strategies to cope with it. Such times can easily be viewed as crisis situations. Following Marlatt (1985), we inform patients that the Chinese character for "crisis" consists of two ideograms, one meaning "danger" and the other "opportunity." Confronting the temptation to use narcotics provides an opportunity to increase self-confidence and the perception of "being in control." This can make it easier to self-manage future episodes of intense pain. In fact, we may suggest that patients cannot fully master the self-management of their chronic pain until they have successfully coped with episodes of intense pain without resorting to mind-altering chemicals.

It is important to keep reiterating the fact that successful coping does not imply gritting one's teeth and bearing unnecessary pain. In our bias against narcotics and other central nervous system depressants, we are not suggesting that there is any virtue in undergoing agony and excessive suffering. Rather, we attempt to reinforce what most chronic patients already know but are sometimes afraid to admit. These drugs are not only poor solutions to chronic pain, but their use tends to create additional problems that only compound the chronic-pain syndrome. Professionals who work with chronic-pain patients know of many individuals who were once narcotic-dependent but then learned to abstain from drug use, not because their pain went away but, rather, because they learned prevention and other constructive ways of coping. Such individuals invariably report that they are better off without narcotics. The process of going from a state of drug dependence to successful self-management is not easy. During the transition period, occurrences of intense pain can be viewed as opportunities to put self-management training to the test. Success during this time significantly reinforces continued self-management.

One obvious stimulus-control procedure, after narcotic reduction has been completed, is to remove all unwanted pain medications from the home environment. As a result, the person would be required to expend some effort contacting a physician to get a prescription unless he or she had easy access to an illegal source of drugs originally prescribed for someone else. Unfortunately, some patients insist on maintaining a supply of drugs at home "in case of emergencies." In such cases, we suggest that before resorting to drug use they try a delay strategy. In other words, an arbitrary temporal delay is self-imposed before giving in to an urge to consume drugs. For example, an individual in intense pain may say to himself, "I really would like to take some codeine right now, but I think I'll hang in there for 15 minutes while I try to relax and divert my attention to something else. When the 15 minutes are up, if I still feel unable to cope on my own, I'll reconsider taking the pill." If the patient successfully manages this period of time, he is in a position to say, "since I made it through those 15 minutes, I'll go another 15 minutes with my self-management techniques and then decide." These delays, with the actual time period determined by the patient, can then be continued until the intense pain crisis is over. This technique forces patients to use self-management techniques rather than resorting to their habitual mode of coping (i.e., using drugs), but only for a limited period of time. The technique also requires them to focus their attention and coping efforts on the immediate present rather than to anticipate a continual build-up in pain intensity to the point that pain becomes absolutely unbearable. Sometimes it is helpful to remind patients that the only pain they really must bear is pain at the present moment. It is the anticipation of future pain that creates anxiety and additional suffering.

If it is believed that analgesics are necessary, patients should be encouraged to use nonnarcotics such as aspirin or acetaminophen on a time-interval basis (e.g., two tablets every 4 hours). Since these drugs do not interfere with cognition, patients can continue using distraction and other cognitive pain-coping strategies. In the event that a patient does give in to the urge to take a narcotic or other mind-altering substance, an attempt should be made to keep this lapse from escalating into a full-blown relapse or a return to the prior level of drug dependency. Since a full description of relapse-prevention procedures is beyond the scope of this book, the reader is referred to the work by Marlatt and Gordon (1985). Although their relapse-prevention model was not developed with chronic-pain patients in mind, it is highly relevant for those who have managed pain with narcotics, alcohol, tranquilizers, and barbiturates.

Patients may need to be reminded repeatedly that our negative bias regarding narcotics and other central nervous system depressants applies only to exacerbations of their chronic pain. Narcotics may be very appropriate for pain associated with acute injuries and disease conditions or severe pain resulting from a malignancy. Consequently, those who fail to make this distinction may feel unnecessarily guilty for receiving narcotic injections following surgery or may subject themselves to unreasonable suffering by refusing narcotics after a serious injury. On the other hand, we know of patients who blamed their physicians for making them redependent on narcotics following routine receipt of such drugs postoperatively.

By practicing good prevention and making use of constructive coping strategies, most chronic-pain patients should be able to manage their pain without use of narcotics, alcohol, tranquilizers, and other central nervous system depressants. One of the most rewarding experiences for professionals in this field is to encounter previously treated chronic-pain patients who were once very dependent on these drugs and then learned to manage pain effectively without them.

SUMMARY

Since many patients undergoing pain-management training report difficulty using nondrug coping strategies during periods of peak pain intensity, it is useful to focus directly on self-management approaches to intense pain episodes. Two general categories are distinguished: preventive strategies and constructive coping strategies that can be used while one is in the midst of intense pain. Prevention involves the identification of potentially controllable pain-intensity triggers. Two areas of prevention are particularly emphasized. Many individuals can prevent chronic-pain exacerbations by modulating their physical activities more carefully. Second, by more effectively managing tension and stressful life demands, one can often prevent increases in pain intensity. Constructive pain-management strategies include behavioral and cognitive coping strategies that do not perpetuate and contribute to the chronic-pain syndrome. They are aimed at reducing, but not necessarily eliminating, sensations of intense pain. Cognitive strategies are particularly emphasized and include attention diversion, self-instructional processes and imagery techniques. The primary goal of this approach to intense pain episodes is to equip pain patients with a variety of self-management "tools" that will give them a greater perception of control over their pain levels. It is also useful to devote special attention to those patients who have been narcotic-dependent. For such individuals, relapse-prevention strategies may be useful.

CHAPTER 7

Managing Stress and Depression

Clinicians working with chronic-pain patients are very aware of the significant degree of situational stress, particularly in the area of interpersonal conflicts, usually experienced by these individuals. Emotional distress is also a significant characteristic of the chronic-pain syndrome. Negative emotional states (e.g., depression, anxiety, and anger) are most certainly the consequence of chronic pain as well as its precursor. Patients can become involved in a destructive cycle in which negative thinking and emotions increase pain perception that, in turn, leads to greater emotional and cognitive distress. The breaking of this cycle is one of the significant challenges facing chronic-pain patients. The present chapter describes the self-management approach to this problem.

COGNITION, STRESS, AND PAIN

Turk et al. (1983) have discussed the relationship between cognitive variables and pain. In reviewing research studies that examined factors differentiating between high and low pain tolerance, they conclude that cognitive processes play a primary role in determining pain perception. Studies have demonstrated that cognitive factors including beliefs, values, expectations, and attributional statements significantly influence pain experience. An individual's belief regarding the cause of a painful sensation, for example, would have considerably different impact if the person believes that the pain is the result of temporary factors rather than a metastatic cancer. Cultural factors such as ethnicity as well as family dynamics greatly influence cognitive style and thus influence an individual's perception of pain. Perhaps most importantly, chronic pain often affects how people view their ability to control many life situations other than physical discomfort, including relationships with significant others, employment options, and the completion of everyday tasks. The sense of self-efficacy in chronic-pain patients is often diminished. Some develop a general negative cognitive set from which most life experiences are viewed as hopeless and futile. Of course, this sense of having little control over life circumstances may have characterized the chronic-pain patient prior to the onset of the pain condition. Whatever the origin, the negativity of chronic-pain patients is well known to those clinicians who work with them. Depression is one obvious outcome of this negative cognitive set.

The relationship between depression and chronic pain has been well documented. Romano and Turner (1985) reviewed research examining the etiological contribution of various factors to this relationship. The most basic explanation of how chronic pain and depression interact is that depression is an obvious outcome of the lifestyle of the chronic-pain patient. Others have theorized that chronic pain is a variant of depressive disorder (Blumer & Heilbronn, 1982). More recently, biochemical links between depression and pain have been suggested as the cause of the close relationship between the two phenomena (France & Krishnan, 1985). Rudy et al. (1988) proposed that depression and pain are related through cognitive mediators that develop as the pain patient becomes more and more limited by his pain. These limitations result in significant feelings of helplessness and reduced self-control that may produce global feelings of worthlessness and futility. Depression results from this interaction among chronic pain, behavioral limitations, and self-deprecatory cognitions.

The cognitive–behavioral view of depression and chronic pain may also account for the high levels of stress found in these patients. In an investigation of the relationship among stress, depression, and chronic pain, Atkinson, Slater, Grant, Patterson, and Garfin (1988) found that depressed mood was the likely factor that linked chronic pain and high levels of life stress. They found that a subgroup of chronic-pain patients who had diagnosable major depression also had significantly higher levels of adverse life events. Nondistressed pain patients had significantly lower levels of depression than did highly stressed patients. The authors also found that distressed chronic-pain patients often experienced their stress in life areas related to their pain condition such as financial problems from being unable to work and multiple hospitalizations. The authors conclude that those chronic-pain patients with both high levels of stress and depression are the ones most likely to be referred to chronic-pain management programs.

Although there are many unanswered questions regarding the interrelationships among stress, depression, and chronic pain, it is clear that the chronic-pain patient is highly susceptible both to feelings of low self-esteem and to high distress. The causal relationships among these three factors are not always clear, but any clinician working with chronic-

pain patients is aware of their close association. In our program, we view
these factors predominantly from a cognitive–behavioral perspective. This
perspective is based on a transactional view of stress and coping (Lazarus
& Folkman, 1984). Losses, threats, challenges, and other stressful demands are cognitively appraised along with available coping alternatives.
Based on this appraisal process, specific coping responses are employed.
Coping efforts may be directed at the perceived problem or at the resulting emotional reactions. These coping responses are influenced, enhanced, or restrained by the various coping resources available to the
individual. Because of the importance placed on appraisal processes,
cognitive therapy has become a significant intervention in our program. In
the next section, we discuss the application of cognitive therapy within the
context of the self-management model.

COGNITIVE THERAPY

Cognitive therapy (CT) is one of the core psychological components in our
program. Of course, much of the foundation of our self-management
model reflects cognitive therapy principles. In all aspects of the program,
we emphasize belief and attitude change as the fundamental process
leading to effective coping with chronic pain. Cognitive therapy allows the
patient to reconceptualize life difficulties, including chronic pain, as solv-
able problems. It focuses on the patient learning a specific schema to
assess and modify irrational, stress-inducing thoughts. In adapting CT to
our program, we identified two goals: (1) to teach patients about the
influence of their thoughts on their emotions and behavior, and (2) to
present a simple formula that patients may use to identify and alter those
irrational thoughts that have often resulted in unpleasant emotions and
poor problem solving. The CT approach we use is similar to that discussed by Ellis (1982) and Beck (1976).

We present the rationale for CT from the very first day of the
program. Although CT may seem simple to the psychologically sophisticated therapist, we have found that it is best to present CT concepts in an
elementary format supplemented by easily understood examples. In introducing CT, we first present patients with the proposition that pain and
stress have a cyclical relationship in which stress increases pain, and
increased pain, in turn, is a stressor. Patients are asked to present personal
examples that illustrate this relationship between stress and pain. Almost
all our patients can immediately provide examples of how stressful life
events have aggravated their pain. It is then pointed out to patients that
their pain could be reduced by improved stress management even when
the underlying physical cause of the pain is unmodifiable. It is also

suggested that patients may benefit from the program even if they do not experience any appreciable pain reduction during treatment. To illustrate this point we often ask patients the following question: "What, if in 3 weeks when you are about to be discharged, your pain level is the same or only slightly less than it is now but you are noticeably less depressed and believe that you are much better able to manage stressful situations in your life? Would you consider the program to be a success?" Patients almost always respond that the program would have been successful for them. By asking the patient this question, we are helping him or her to understand the important interrelationship among thoughts, stress, and pain. They must see that physical pain is only one source of their suffering. Other sources of distress in their lives are separate from pain and are within their ability to manage. Some patients argue that pain is the only really negative aspect in their lives and that it is the sole cause of their distress. It takes only minimal intervention to help these individuals to recognize that other factors, although they are perhaps aggravated by the pain, are upsetting them. Pain is but one stressor among many others.

A patient, for example, may say that he and his wife are not getting along because the pain prevents him from helping around the house. He has concluded, therefore, that pain is the sole cause of marital arguments and his resulting anger and depression. The fallacy of this conclusion can be pointed out by asking the patient whether he and his wife ever argued before he developed a pain condition. In descriptions of these arguments, a pattern emerges that reveals the patient to be extremely sensitive to criticism from his wife, no matter how minuscule the problem may be. He responds to her in a defensive, confrontational manner that soon leads to a loud, nonproductive argument. It is clear that this same communication pattern continues in the present when the patient, being in chronic pain, is especially sensitive to any suggestion that he is less than perfect. By discussing this example, we can illustrate the critical point that the problem that led to his frustration and depression was not just pain but rather a destructive pattern of communication between him and his wife that had existed prior to the development of the pain problem.

We often use another illustration with patients to assist them in understanding that they could feel better even if their pain condition remained the same. A circle is drawn on the board with a line through it about one-quarter of the way down from the top. The circle represents the patient's life experience in the present. In the smaller, upper part of the circle, a plus sign is drawn, and in the larger, bottom part a negative sign is drawn. The + symbol represents positive emotional feelings in the patient's life and the − symbol represents negative feelings. Patients new to the program often agree that a much smaller percentage of their life is positive, and the larger percentage of their time is negative. They are asked whether they would consider the program to be a success if the percentages in the two parts of the circle could be made equal or even reversed. They usually respond "yes" with certainty. This example helps patients understand the important cognitive principle of the relativity of positive and negative feelings and situations. They can begin to realize that their lives were never free of all suffering before their pain condition and never would have been had they never suffered from chronic pain. Thus, much of their recent unhappiness is the result of unrealistic expectations of themselves leading to frustration, anger, and depression. Patients have to see the value of relative improvement in order to experience benefit from self-management. With these above examples fully discussed and their points understood, patients are ready to move on to the specifics of CT.

The first sessions of CT are didactic and emphasize many of the principles discussed above. In discussing the relationship between stress and pain, we use specific examples of how people often blame situations for their negative emotions. A commonly used excuse from an actual patient example follows:

> K.L., a 50-year-old chronic-pain patient, blamed his almost daily headaches on "stupid, crummy drivers" on the freeway, especially during the afternoon rush hour. In particular, he was most upset with drivers who followed his car too closely. He usually coped with these drivers in one of three ways. First, he sometimes braked suddenly in the hope that the driver behind him would get scared or even get hurt. Second, he purposely cut behind the other driver and followed him too closely. Third, he sometimes drove in the lane next to the other driver and nudged that car into the next lane or onto the freeway shoulder. When asked what emotion he was feeling as this situation developed, K.L. readily acknowledged that he was feeling anger. However when asked *why* he was angry, he emphatically stated that it was because of the other driver. In effect, K.L. told us that he had no choice but to react the way he did (i.e., "when people drive like that I'm naturally going to get angry. No one is going to push me around like that.").

At this point we begin to diagram the example as follows:

    A = the situation: the other driver following too closely
    C = the emotion: anger
    D = behavioral reactions: three examples of reckless driving

It is pointed out to patients that K.L. believed that A caused C, which led to D. If this were true, we would almost never have control over life events, our emotions, or our behavior. We would simply react to what others do to us, making us puppets on a string. Patients will readily agree that we have little direct control over many common stressful situations (e.g., fellow workers, ex-spouses, paying taxes, bureaucratic paperwork) and that in dealing with these situations we often experience unpleasant emotions. When we feel these emotions, we rarely cope effectively with the situations that have made us feel this way.

Then, returning to the example of K.L., patients are asked how they might have reacted to the freeway tailgater. Most patients respond with a cooler head than did K.L. They are then asked what is different about how they were able to react versus the behavior of K.L. Patients will list an assortment of different interpretations of the situation than did K.L. One patient may say that he would be concerned about the other driver and would move over immediately. Another patient may say to himself, "sooner or later the tailgater will move over so I'll just stay in my lane and not worry about it." A third patient might suggest that the driver is in a hurry to get to an important business meeting. None of these three alternative interpretations would make one as upset as K.L.'s overly hostile reaction to the bad driver. More importantly, none of these thoughts would lead to the negative, potentially dangerous, coping behaviors used by K.L. Through examples such as this, patients can begin to understand that a person's thoughts about situations determine his or her emotional and behavioral response to a particular situation. We then introduce the letter B into our diagram as follows:

A = the situation
B = cognitive interpretation of the situation
C = consequent emotional reactions
D = coping responses

B is presented as the true cause of negative emotions and poor coping. Patients are also reminded that in the K.L. example it was K.L. who suffered from stress and increased pain and probably not the other driver. In this instance, the patient's irrational thoughts increased the likelihood of his suffering and provided him with little demonstrable reward.

Simple examples, such as the K.L. case, which demonstrates how interpretations of everyday events affect our emotional health, can serve as an excellent introduction to CT. It clearly shows how these interpretations are relative and vary from individual to individual. Certain thoughts lead to productive coping, whereas other thoughts may lead to unnecessary depression, anxiety, and anger. Patients benefit from understanding that they cannot directly control their emotions or their behavior in any lasting, substantial way without first changing their thoughts. This process of reviewing habitual thought patterns fits well into the self-management model, since the patient is the best person to monitor his own thoughts. The patient must be reminded that the CT process is ongoing and reflects a coping, rather than curative, perspective. No one ever thinks rationally all the time, nor would that be a reasonable goal for anyone. Thus, CT aims at identifying and changing recurrent irrational thought patterns that cause chronic negative emotions.

The specific focus of the CT groups is on learning to identify irrational ways of thinking or "cognitive distortions." We use a list of 15 such distortions adapted from McKay, Davis, and Fanning (1981). Examples of these irrational ways of thinking include filtering, catastrophizing, and "shoulds." Generally, these distortions are similar to ones discussed in many previous works by Beck, Rush, Shaw, and Emery (1979), Burns (1980), Ellis and Harper (1975), and Lazarus and Fay (1975). Each distortion is discussed, and patients are asked to identify the ones that they use. Patients are encouraged to realize that they can exercise some control over their emotional health by altering the way they think. Everyday examples of stressful events are analyzed in terms of how these could be interpreted differently so as to minimize their stressful impact and maximize use of adaptive coping responses. Most importantly, we attempt to help patients reconceptualize chronic pain as one "A" (i.e., situation) in their life that they can respond differently to, both emotionally and behaviorally, if they think differently about it. Thus, pain is put into a new perspective, making it one of many life stresses as opposed to the overwhelming life burden that is the cause of all the patient's misery. The message becomes clear: Even pain can be thought about differently—in a way that facilitates successful coping rather than depression and withdrawal.

As is true throughout the psychological parts of our program, patients begin to focus less and less on pain as the days pass. In CT group, we usually focus more on stressful relationships, work problems, and frustrations in dealing with the medical and disability bureaucracy. The following example of a problem discussed in CT will illustrate the therapeutic process:

M.N. was a 40-year-old patient with 15 years of chronic low back pain. He had a stable marriage of 18 years and two teen-aged children. During the second week of the CT group, he identified a stressful situation at work that contributed to his often angry demeanor. His frustration at work created tension at home and aggravated his pain. M.N. worked as a typesetter for a large printing company. He had worked there for almost 20 years developing an efficient routine that had given him shop seniority and job security. He planned to take an early retirement at age 45. Seven months prior to entering the program, M.N. was assigned an assistant who happened to be a nephew of the company's owner. The assistant was on 1 year's probation, as were all new employees. He was learning different aspects of the printing business and was to work under M.N. for 3 more months. The new employee was young and not a good worker. He took shortcuts that upset M.N.'s work routine. When he messed up the printing machines, M.N. took it upon himself to clean up after him. M.N. was angry throughout the day but did not feel that he could complain because of the man's family connection to the business. He felt extremely tense at work and often yelled at his wife and children when he arrived home each evening.

When introduced to CT, M.N. could see no relevance of the therapeutic principles to this situation. He believed that these problems were caused by another person over whom he had no control. We helped him to identify a number of distortions in the way he thought about this situation. First, he *catastrophized* about work continuously, thinking that he would never be able to go back to his old, comfortable routine. Second, he was *filtering* by focusing on one negative aspect of his job to the exclusion of the remaining positive aspects. Third, he was failing to understand the ways he could exercise *control* in this situation. M.N. accepted this feedback slowly and began to understand that his distorted thinking had resulted in anxiety, depression, and anger. These negative emotions lead to poor coping that had negatively affected his job, his family, and his pain.

We worked to identify rational alternative statements that could counter each of the distorted thoughts. In response to catastrophizing, M.N. reminded himself that the assistant would be leaving in a few more months; by focusing on the temporary nature of his assignment, M.N. did not become as upset. To stop filtering, he concentrated on those aspects of his job he still enjoyed. Much of the day, it turned out, the assistant was not even with him. M.N. liked his job, and when he completed a project, he felt a great deal of satisfaction. He was still finishing all of his responsibilities even during the time that he had to supervise the co-worker. Focusing on the remaining positive elements of his work left him feeling good about work. In discussing the control issue, M.N. was encouraged to identify as many actions as possible, no matter how small they seemed, that could be used to change the work situation. Some of these alternatives were more risky than others (e.g., quitting his job), and M.N. rejected them. Certain changes, however, were realistic. He could assign the worker to another employee part of the time. He could informally talk to his supervisor about the situation. He also realized that he had been treating the owner's nephew too softly and had not really done a very good job of teaching him the printing business. His own fear of criticizing the boss's nephew, although not totally unrealistic, had been carried too far, and he had lost sight of his own excellent work record, his job seniority, and union protection from unfair treatment if the boss did become angry with him about how he handled his nephew. Of course, these distortions identified in this specific situation were not simply isolated examples for M.N. Catastrophizing, focusing on the negative, and feeling no control in situations were all attitudes that had characterized this patient's perception of many life demands. He was encouraged to challenge himself whenever he felt depressed, angry, or anxious and identify how those feelings were tied to his thoughts and were not the result of people or circumstances outside of his control. M.N. also began to understand, as the group sessions continued, that in thinking in the distorted ways that produced stress he was the one who suffered emotionally and physically. He came to realize that his habitual thought patterns were his greatest source of stress and that blaming others would only lead to frustration, depression, and anger.

As part of the CT approach we introduce the patients to the concept of "rational comebacks" (McKay et al., 1981). Patients are encouraged to develop self-statements that reflect rational responses to identified distorted thoughts. For example, if a patient became aware that he was overfocusing on personal losses to the point of being chronically depressed (i.e., "filtering"), he could use the rational comeback, "I need to shift my focus to situations in my life that have gone well and not magnify my difficult situations out of proportion." Rational comebacks are self-statements that the patient can use to modify irrational thoughts. We spend considerable time with patients helping them to generate effective rational responses to counter their distortions. Patients are asked to focus on how using these rational statements has relatively immediate emotional benefits in that they find themselves feeling better and focusing on more positive aspects of their life. In addition, as the patients feel more positive they are better able to develop solutions to the real problems that they must face. This process of identifying distortions, generating rational comebacks, feeling more positive, and learning more effective coping behaviors is a cyclical process that we hope will become reinforcing and self-perpetuating.

We have found CT to be a highly effective intervention with many chronic-pain patients. It provides them with a relatively simple scheme for analyzing and resolving their own problems as the self-management model encourages. Further, CT reinforces for patients the awareness of their own responsibility for their well-being. It also shows the patient that how one copes with stress has a direct impact on the experience of chronic pain. Although we have a separate CT group in our program, the basic premise of CT is continuously stressed throughout the entire program. Patients are told of the importance of continuing the CT process after the inpatient phase of the program. They are given written materials that they may refer to during and after the program as a reminder of CT principles and examples of distorted thinking.

DISCOVERING MORE EFFECTIVE WAYS OF COPING WITH DEPRESSION AND STRESS

In addition to helping patients identify and modify distorted perceptions of stressful situations, it is important to help them discover more effective ways of coping. Coping efforts can be directed at either the presumed source of the problem (problem-focused coping) or at the distressing emotions (emotion-focused coping). Both types of coping are important, although one may be more appropriate than the other depending on the situation.

Problem-Focused Coping

Two general problem-focused coping frameworks may be introduced. First is the utilization of effective problem-solving skills using the methods described by D'Zurilla (1986). According to this view, an individual's difficulty in coping with a seemingly unsolvable problem is a failure correctly to define and find reasonable solutions to the specific problem. This perspective is in contrast to the futility and helplessness expressed by depressed patients when they are faced with difficult, challenging problems. D'Zurilla and Goldfried (1971) developed a five-step approach that guides the patient through a process of problem identification and the listing and evaluation of alternative solutions for those problems. Specific problems presented by group participants are used to illustrate the value of this procedure. This general approach to problem-solving skills complements CT, described above, in that it views stressful situations as within the coping capacity of individuals depending on their attitudes, beliefs, and expectations.

Another problem-focused coping approach emphasizes effective communication skills. Assertive action, in contrast to passive or aggressive behavior, is of value to many of our pain patients, who often alternate between nonexpression of feelings and angry confrontations with others. By means of lectures, discussion, written handouts, and role playing, patients are introduced to the general principles of assertiveness training (Alberti & Emmons, 1982). Particular emphasis is placed on helping patients respond more assertively in pain-related situations. For example, many of our patients interact ineffectively with physicians and bureaucratic disability agencies. They often do not pose the questions they actually want to ask of health-care workers and alternate between a passive stance and an angry, aggressive posture with these authority figures. The patients leave such interactions frustrated and view their passivity or temper outbursts as further proof of their worthlessness. Patients in such situations can benefit from learning to interact assertively by being prepared with written questions for their physicians, asking for clarification of responses when experts use complex medical or legal terminology, and assuming a persistent but not overbearing stance toward health-care givers.

Assertion skills are also important when one is interacting with family and friends. Those patients who tend to be very hostile and demanding are encouraged to express their needs and desires in a more appropriate, assertive manner that recognizes and respects the rights of others. Patients are also taught to express their feelings and needs more directly rather than communicating them through pain behavior. They are taught to take the initiative in assertively informing family and friends of more helpful ways of responding to displays of pain. For example, frequent inquiries regarding the patient's pain condition and overly solicitous responses are less helpful than efforts to divert the patient's attention away from pain. As mentioned in Chapter 4, self-management of physical activities may require the patient to request help assertively when he or she must perform a demanding physical task or to refuse requests by another person to engage in a physical task that may exacerbate the pain condition.

Communication is also presented as an important means of combating depression. A common component of the depressed cycle is social withdrawal and noncommunication with significant others. As the person becomes more self-absorbed and preoccupied, depressive cognitions multiply. Problems appear increasingly burdensome and unsolvable. Consequently, depressed patients are encouraged to share their thoughts with family members, trusted friends, or a professional counselor. In group or individual counseling sessions, we encourage depressed, noncommunicative patients to open up. The mere process of increased communication to a caring, empathetic individual is therapeutic to some degree. More important, it can enable depressed patients to receive feedback regarding distorted cognitions, clarification or redefinition of their problems, and to develop a more realistic perspective regarding coping alternatives. With some chronic-pain patients we discover a long history of a previously undiagnosed depressive disorder that preceded onset of the pain condition. As is discussed in Chapter 9, such patients may require psychotherapy in addition to self-management training.

Emotion-Focused Coping

For some of our patients, emotion-focused coping begins with increased awareness of their emotions. Associated with the excessive somatic focus of many chronic-pain patients is a failure to recognize some common feelings. This is particularly common among our male veteran patients who have been socialized to deny or inhibit depression and anxiety. Such feelings may be considered signs of weakness or unmanliness.

It is also important that patients understand that negative emotions are not necessarily the result of distorted thinking. Anxiety, fear, sadness, and anger are normal and inevitable responses to many life events. It may be important to learn how to discriminate between healthy and unhealthy expressions of these emotional states. In addition to cognitive appraisal, effective problem solving, and assertive action, patients are encouraged to develop more effective ways of coping with their negative emotions. Two general self-management frameworks are presented. The first is the importance of constructive action in spite of the presence of negative emotions. The second is the use of healthy relaxation strategies to cope with emotions accompanied by increased tension (i.e., fear, anxiety, and anger). Since relaxation approaches are discussed at length in the next section, we focus here on the use of constructive action.

Constructive action is perhaps best seen as an effective response to depression. Referring to the general biopsychosocial model discussed in Chapter 3, patients are taught to view depression as involving an interaction among emotional, mental, behavioral, and even physiological elements. Once depressed affect takes hold, irrespective of the cause, the person's physiology, thoughts, and behaviors are all influenced in a way that reinforces and perpetuates the depression. In particular, thinking tends to become distorted, and activity diminishes. Physiologically, the person may experience loss of energy, fatigue, appetite changes, and a variety of unpleasant somatic sensations. Vicious cycles are created that serve to maintain the depression. It then becomes extremely difficult to modify directly one's depressed mood, negative thoughts, distortions, and associated physiological sensations. The greatest possibility for change is in the action component. Unfortunately, most depressed people do not want to *do* anything because they do not *feel* like doing anything. It is as though they are waiting to feel better (i.e., not depressed) before they can engage in constructive action.

Constructive action as a response to depression may be approached from the perspective of Morita therapy principles (Reynolds, 1984). Reynolds has described Morita and other Japanese forms of psychotherapy in numerous books. Along with some behavioral approaches, Morita therapy emphasizes action as the principal way of managing negative feelings. People who focus excessively on their feelings become unable to live productively. Patients are encouraged to concentrate on behavioral goals. Feelings are viewed as ephemeral phenomena that are too changeable to form the basis of individual behavior. Therapy is aimed at helping individuals identify paths to life goals and to encourage patients to ignore feelings that would interfere with the behaviors necessary to reach these goals. Morita therapy encourages focusing on the world outside the individual and emphasizes that pleasure in life is the result of productive activity. Morita principles have some obvious similarities to certain fundamental ideas of cognitive–behavioral theory including its emphasis on problem solving, identifying purposeful (i.e., coping) behaviors, and de-emphasis of trying to alter negative emotional states directly. Morita therapy also strongly encourages a rational, realistic appraisal of situations that is strikingly similar to what is found in the writings of cognitive–behavioral theorists such as Ellis (1982) and Burns (1980). We have found that the constructive action perspective encouraged by Morita therapy adapts well to the self-management approach to chronic pain.

RELAXATION TRAINING AND TENSION MANAGEMENT

Early in the program, we discuss the relationship between tension and pain. It is pointed out that tension can be manifested both physiologically (e.g., increased muscle tension, autonomic arousal) and by negative thoughts associated with worry, frustration, irritation, regret, etc. Three sources of tension are distinguished. First, pain itself is a source of tension. Second, the consequences of coping with a chronic-pain condition are often stressful. Examples of such consequences include disability and unemployment, financial problems, and conflicts with doctors and the disability compensation system. Third, tension can result from various demands and hassles of daily life that have nothing to do with the pain condition. These are demands and annoyances that can be experienced by anyone. In each case, the resulting tension can contribute to the amount of pain experienced.

It is also emphasized that tension per se is not the problem. Tension is both normal and necessary in order to meet challenges and accomplish many tasks. The problem is excess tension. Excess occurs when there is more tension than necessary to meet a particular demand or accomplish a given task. The physiological, mental, and emotional consequences of excess tension can amplify pain and suffering. Compounding the problem is the fact that the presence of excess tension may not be consciously recognized.

Patients are introduced to the idea of a tension–relaxation continuum, as illustrated on the top of page 153. At one end is a state of extreme physical and mental tension; at the opposite extreme is a state of deep relaxation. We can arbitrarily assign the number 100 to the high-tension end and a 0 to the deep-relaxation end. Deep relaxation should not be equated with sleep, since people are not necessarily deeply relaxed while sleeping. During the course of a day, people fluctuate somewhere between these two extremes. There is no single point on this scale that is ideal. A "desirable" level of tension is relative to what needs to be accomplished. It

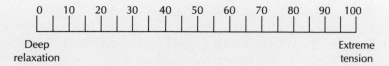

is impossible to accomplish most tasks at either extreme. Extreme states of tension tend to disrupt and interfere with one's ability to cope with most demands, whereas when in a state of deep relaxation, one does not have the energy to accomplish anything.

Patients are then introduced to the idea of relaxation as one way of countering excess tension. Three types of relaxation are distinguished: coping relaxation, time-out relaxation, and relaxing activities.

Coping Relaxation

This type of relaxation is aimed at helping people cope more effectively with stressful situations and episodes of emotional distress or intense pain. It is meant to be used anywhere and at any time. The particular method we use is called the "signal breath." It consists of a relatively deep inhalation that is held for a few moments and then released slowly. Just at the moment the breath is released, the person is instructed to say to himself a relevant cue word or phrase such as "relax," "let go," "cool it," or "easy does it." During this process an attempt is also made to scan quickly and then release areas of excessive muscle tension as the breath is being exhaled. Common target areas for increased tension include the face, neck, and shoulders. The entire process takes only a few seconds. It has much in common with the "quieting reflex" (QR) discussed by Stroebel (1983).

In addition to helping the person experience an immediate sense of tension release, the signal breath is aimed at disrupting habitual and automatic response tendencies that interfere with effective coping. We inform patients that coping relaxation is not meant to discharge all tension, nor is it meant to solve the problem that evoked the tension in the first place. Rather, it serves as a signal or reminder to stop and think. By lowering tension to even a small degree, one may be in a better position to think more clearly and act more wisely. When pausing to think in the midst of a stressful situation or time of emotional distress, one might consider some of the following questions:

1. What am I feeling right now?
2. What is the situation or event that has triggered these feelings?
3. Am I viewing this situation clearly, or am I distorting it?
4. Can I do anything right now to change this situation, or do I need to focus primarily on managing my feelings?

5. What can I do right now to cope with these feelings?

The signal breath can also be a useful preparation for coping with an intense pain episode. The following questions may be considered:

1. Can I identify the immediate cause or trigger for this increased pain?
2. What positive actions (physical and mental) can I take right now that will help me to survive this temporary episode of increased pain?

Patients are instructed to look for opportunities to use the signal breath. Subsequent group sessions can then be used to discuss specific situations in which this coping relaxation technique was applied. Ultimately, the goal is to make coping relaxation a habitual response to episodes of increased tension and pain.

Time-Out Relaxation

The second approach to relaxation requires one to take time out from ordinary activities and spend time (e.g., 5 to 30 minutes) doing a special relaxation procedure. Unlike coping relaxation, this approach requires one to find a quiet environment to reduce external distractions. This enables the person to devote full attention to relaxing the mind and body as deeply as possible. Referring to the tension–relaxation continuum, it is pointed out that with time-out relaxation procedures it is possible to achieve deeper states of relaxation.

The purpose and benefits of time-out relaxation for those with chronic pain should be carefully spelled out. Drawing from Turk et al. (1983), we point out that relaxation can accomplish the following:

1. Relax tense muscles. Muscle tension resulting from the pain itself or from emotional stress often increases painful sensations. Therefore, relaxation reduces the amount of pain that is directly caused by tense muscles.

2. Attention diversion relaxation exercises require one to direct attention to pleasant sensations, thoughts, and images. Although one still may feel the pain to some extent, one cannot be fully attentive to one's pain and at the same time direct one's attention to relaxing thoughts and sensations. Thus, by occupying one's attention with something else, relaxation reduces the amount of pain a person experiences.

3. Awareness of tension. Many individuals are tense without being aware of it. Also some people may think they are relaxed when actually they are not. By practicing time-out relaxation and experiencing what it feels like to really "let go" and become deeply relaxed, a person also learns to become more aware of his or her own subtle signs of physical and mental tension. By becoming more aware of tension throughout the day, one can learn to use those signs of tension as cues or reminders to use coping relaxation.

4. Help with sleep problems. Many people with chronic pain have difficulties with sleep. Consequently, a person may find it harder to cope with pain when he or she is tired. Time-out relaxation can help by making it easier to fall asleep or by serving as a restful substitute for sleep.

In addition to presenting a rationale for time-out relaxation, we point out the following. In order to benefit from time-out relaxation, one must use it regularly. Deep relaxation is a skill, and like any other skill, it has be learned. For some people this comes easily; for others, it takes longer and requires much more practice. It is important that one be patient with oneself and not always expect immediate, significant results. It is easiest to learn relaxation initially under more ideal circumstances. For example, if a person wanted to learn how to swim, he or she would not start off in deep, rough water; rather, it would be better to start off in the shallow end of a swimming pool. Thus, one should first practice relaxation in a quiet environment, and at times when one is less likely to be interrupted, less tense, and experiencing less pain. Most people find it difficult to concentrate on relaxation when they are tired, tense, emotionally upset, or are experiencing intense pain. Later, as patients become more skilled at relaxation, they may be able to use it at more difficult times.

In addition to a quiet environment, Benson (1975) lists three other requirements for achieving time-out relaxation ("relaxation response"). First, it is helpful to be in a comfortable position. Traditional meditative postures (e.g., sitting in a cross-legged position) are not practical for most of our patients. Since some patients complain that no position is completely comfortable, we instruct them to find the most comfortable position possible under the present circumstances. Some prefer to do time-out relaxation while reclining in bed. We inform them that the bed is usually not the best place to learn time-out relaxation because of one's tendency to fall asleep. On the other hand, if patients are using this form of relaxation to facilitate sleep onset, this is permissible. For training purposes, we have our patients sit in soft high-backed chairs with adequate lumbar support. Most of our patients have reclining chairs that can be used for their home practice. We then describe some of the typical behavioral features of a relaxed person (Poppen, 1988). For example, we may tell them the following:

A relaxed person sits in a chair with both feet flat on the ground. If one is seated on a recliner with a leg extender, the feet are pointed away from each other at a comfortable angle. The torso, hips, and legs are straight in the chair. The shoulders are rounded and at the same height. Hands and lower arms are resting on the lap or on the arms of the chair. The hands and fingers are uncrossed and are curled in a claw-like fashion. The head and neck are supported by the back of the chair and are in a relatively straight line. The eyes are gently closed, the face appears loose, the jaw is slack, and the lips are slightly parted. Very little movement is observed other than the abdomen and chest rising and falling slowly and regularly with each breath cycle. No sounds can be heard from the nose or throat while the person is breathing.

Since some of our patients initially have very poor sitting tolerance, we inform them that it is permissible to shift their position during the relaxation exercises. However, they should try to maintain the state of relaxation as best as possible as they change positions.

Another aspect of time-out relaxation involves a mental process. This refers to some object of attentional focus that facilitates relaxation. The mind may be directed to an external object or sound, to various parts of one's body, to a rhythmic body function such as breathing, a repetitive word or phrase, or to relaxing mental imagery. We point out that there is no single relaxation technique that is best for everyone. Consequently, we expose our patients to a variety of relaxation methods and suggest that they adopt an experimental attitude to determine which techniques work best. We also believe that it is a good idea to determine beforehand whether any group participants have had prior exposure or training in methods of relaxation or meditation. Those who have had prior exposure can then be questioned about their experiences and expectations regarding time-out relaxation.

We usually begin training with a simple breathing-awareness exercise. There are several variations in using breathing exercises for time-out relaxation. Most approaches involve instructions in slow, deep, abdominal breathing (e.g., McCaffery, 1979). We have also used "noninterference" methods that involve attention to natural breathing processes. The following is a sample of a script that we have used:

To begin with, just take in a deep breath and hold it . . . hold it until you notice tension developing in your chest . . . and then let the air out slowly, relaxing as you do so. Close your eyes and take in another deep breath . . . once again hold it until tension starts building up . . . and then relax; let go completely. As you let your breathing return now to a normal, natural rhythm, simply become aware of your breathing . . . direct your mind to your breathing . . . pay close attention to your breathing by noticing each and every breath . . . just watch it . . . without trying to change, without trying to interfere . . . becoming aware of how easily your body breathes itself . . . automatically . . . all the time, whether asleep or awake, aware or unaware . . . constantly breathing . . . and all you have to do right now is to watch and be aware . . . paying close attention to the natural rhythm of your breath . . . allowing the breath to be as it is. If it is slow, let it be slow. If it is deep, let it be deep. If it is shallow, let it be shallow. Just let your breath be natural and free . . . let go completely . . . just be aware of the sensation as the breath enters . . . and then leaves your nostrils . . . notice what it feels like as the breath flows in . . . and out . . . in . . . and out . . . notice the slight pause between each inhalation . . . and exhalation . . . be aware of the natural expansion . . . and contraction of your lungs with each breath flowing in . . . and out . . . notice how this causes your chest to rise and fall ever so slightly. Perhaps also noticing your abdomen rising . . . and falling each time you breathe in . . . and out. Experience the natural tides of your breath, the ebb . . . and flow, as it comes . . . and goes, in . . . and out, that natural rhythm . . . no need to change, nothing to hold onto, nothing to do . . . just awareness . . . watching . . . observing . . . and allowing . . . the continual flow of your body breathing itself . . . easily . . . and naturally. And as you continue watching your body . . . breathing itself, you may begin to discover that each time you exhale, each time you breathe out, you are becoming more relaxed . . . more comfortable . . . and more at ease. With each breath cycle, feeling yourself, experiencing yourself becoming more and more deeply relaxed. And for the next several minutes you can continue this awareness on your own . . . keeping your awareness on your breathing . . . and even if your attention wanders, or is distracted, you can just bring it back . . . over and over again to your breathing . . . continuing on your own until I remind you when to stop. [Silence] And now you can begin to bring your awareness back to a more normal, alert, and wide-awake state . . . at the count of 3 . . . beginning with 1 . . . 2 . . . 3, opening your eyes and feeling so refreshed.

Patients are then given instructions for practicing a focused breathing exercise on their own. Various methods for keeping attention focused on breath cycles are suggested (e.g., counting breath cycles, visualizing expansion and contraction of the lungs, observing the abdomen rising and falling). Patients can be instructed to pair the word "relax" with each exhalation.

After introducing focused breathing, we turn to passive body-awareness approaches. These exercises are patterned after the autogenic therapy procedures originally developed by Schultz and Luthe (1969). They involve directing attention to various parts of the body along with suggests of relaxation. The following is a sample script:

Begin by assuming a comfortable position in your chair. Notice how the chair is supporting your body. Just allow your body to become relaxed and heavy as though you are sinking into the chair. Allow all of your muscles to become loose and limp as a rag doll. Now focus your attention on your left hand . . . Just think about your left hand, tuning in to the feelings from it . . . Don't worry if your attention wanders. If it does, just bring it back to your left hand. And as you think about your left hand, you may notice the muscles in it becoming loose and limp . . . as if the tension is just flowing out of your fingers and dissolving . . . allowing your hand to become relaxed and soft, loose and limp. And then the relaxation can begin to work its way slowly up your left arm . . . past your wrist and into your forearm. Let the muscles of your forearm become loose and limp. Feel the gentle relaxation flowing through the muscles of your forearm . . . past your elbow and into your upper arm . . . as the relaxation moves from muscle to muscle . . . penetrating deeply and dissolving the tension. . . . Let your entire left arm become loose, limp, heavy, and relaxed. Letting go is voluntary, pleasantly under your control . . . There's no effort involved . . . All you have to do is just tune in to your arm and watch it happen . . . noticing your left arm growing more and more relaxed . . . and now including your left shoulder as the gentle relaxation penetrates into your shoulder, loosening the muscles, dissolving the tension . . . feeling your shoulder becoming heavy, loose, and relaxed . . . more and more deeply relaxed. . . . And now tune in to your right hand. Think about your right hand and allow the muscles to become loose and limp. Feel the relaxation flowing through your fingers and hand, as the muscles of your hand are becoming soft, loose, relaxed, and heavy. And as the relaxation flows past your wrist and into your forearm, you can feel your forearm becoming looser . . . heavier . . . more and more relaxed. And now let it flow in to your upper arm . . . relaxing the muscles of your upper arm . . . feeling your entire right arm become more and more relaxed . . . notice the pleasant relaxation penetrating the muscles of your shoulder . . . as your right shoulder is becoming loose and limp . . . heavy and relaxed . . . more and more relaxed. And as the relaxation grows and deepens in both arms, you may notice your entire body becoming more relaxed . . . as you continue to breathe freely and easily . . . with each gentle breath you can sink even more deeply into relaxation, allowing your body to feel more comfortable . . . heavy and relaxed. Let the relaxation now flow up the back of your neck, dissolving any tension . . . noticing your neck muscles becoming loose and slack . . . relaxed and comfortable. And then let this relaxation continue to flow up the back of your head . . . spreading out across your scalp. . . . Feel the relaxation flowing through your scalp to the sides of your head . . . the top of your head . . . letting that pleasant relaxation smooth out your scalp . . . including your forehead . . . and your eyes . . . as your eyes remain gently closed . . . allow the muscles of your eyes to become relaxed . . . noticing the relaxation spreading throughout your face . . . including your mouth and tongue . . . allow your jaw to become loose and slack . . . and all the muscles of your face becoming loose and limp . . . soft and relaxed . . . growing more deeply relaxed. And now

allow the pleasant feeling of relaxation to move down into your chest . . . spreading out across your chest . . . loosening the muscles with each relaxing breath you take . .
  it's so easy to let go . . . and each time the air goes out, you may notice yourself sinking even more deeply into relaxation . . . noticing how pleasant it feels to be so relaxed and yet awake . . . and aware of your body becoming heavier, more relaxed and more comfortable . . .

This type of relaxation patter continues to include other areas of the body such as the abdomen, back, hips, buttocks, upper legs, knees, lower legs, ankles, and feet. There are many variations of passive body-awareness relaxation exercises. Some are more repetitive and are stated in the first person (e.g., "My right hand is heavy and warm . . . my right hand is heavy and warm . . . my right arm is heavy and warm . . . my right arm is heavy and warm . . .").Other examples of passive body-awareness relaxation exercises are found in Shealy (1977) and Mason (1980).

Unlike many others who teach relaxation to chronic-pain patients, we tend not to use progressive muscle-relaxation procedures. This approach to relaxation requires the person to first tense specific muscles and then let them relax (Bernstein & Borkovec, 1973; Bernstein & Given, 1984; McGuigan, 1984). Since our patients often complained that their pain increased when they tensed various muscles, we tend to use the more passive approaches described above. Furthermore, we are aware of no solid evidence for the superiority of progressive muscle relaxation over other time-out relaxation procedures.

As discussed in Chapter 5, we also introduce patients to external-focus relaxation approaches. This may involve attention to a visual object or to sounds. Patients are guided through several examples of these approaches. We then encourage them to experiment on their own and identify specific environmental stimuli (e.g., works of art, photographs, nature sounds, or types of music) that are the most conducive to a relaxing state.

Finally, we introduce patients to relaxation imagery. After discussing what mental imagery is and how it can facilitate relaxation, we expose patients to some guided relaxation-imagery exercises. The following is an example of one of the scripts we have used:

Picture yourself right now in a log cabin somewhere high up in the mountains. . . . It's wintertime, but even though it is very cold outside, you can enjoy the comfort of being in that cabin . . . for inside of the cabin is a large fireplace with a brightly blazing fire providing plenty of heat and warmth . . . and now you can go up to one of the windows and notice the frost on the windowpane . . . you can even put your warm hand on the cold, hard glass of the windowpane feeling the heat from your hand and fingers melting the frost. . . . And then to get a view of the outside, you can begin to open the window, feeling it give way against the pressure of your hand; as the window opens, you take a big breath of that pure, fresh, cool mountain air and feel so good. Looking outside you can see the snow on the ground and lots of tall evergreen trees. And then looking off in the distance and seeing a wonderful view . . . perhaps of a valley down below or other mountain peaks far, far in the distance. . . . And now you can close the window and walk over to the fire feeling its warmth as you get closer. . . . Go ahead and sit back in a comfortable chair facing the fire . . . or if you wish, you can lie down next to the fire on a soft bearskin rug . . . feeling the soothing warmth of the fire against your skin . . . letting your body absorb the warmth bringing deep relaxation and comfort. . . . You can also enjoy looking at the fire, seeing the burning logs, hearing the crackling of the logs and hissing sound from the sap encountering the fire . . . smelling the fragrant smoke from the burning logs. You can even look around noticing the room as it is illuminated by the light from the fire . . . noticing the flickering shadows on the walls . . . noticing the furniture and any other objects in the room . . . just look around and take it all in . . . all the sights and sounds and smells . . . feeling so peaceful in this place . . . so calm and completely tranquil. And you can be reminded that even though the cold wind is howling outside, you can feel so warm and comfortable inside . . . letting that comfort spread to all parts of your mind. And in this place you have absolutely nothing to worry about . . . for all that really matters is that you just allow yourself to enjoy the peacefulness, enjoy the deep comfort of being in this place right now . . . as a relaxed, drowsy feeling comes over you . . . and all the sights and sounds and smells gradually fade far away . . . while you drift . . . and float and dream in that cabin far off in the mountains. (Pause) And now, whenever you are ready, you can bring yourself back to a normal, alert, and wide-awake state by counting slowly from 1 to 3, so that when you reach the number 3 you will open your eyes feeling completely refreshed and comfortable.

When using guided relaxation imagery, it is important to emphasize that it is not necessary that patients follow the scene exactly as presented. Guided imagery is used more to illustrate the process. Thus, patients should feel free to modify the images according to their own preference. Guidelines for the use of imagery are discussed more fully by Kroger and Fezler (1976) and McCaffery (1979). Kroger and Fezler (1976) also present many specific examples of guided images from their hypnobehavioral therapy framework. Ultimately the goal in self-management is for patients to develop their own relaxing imagery.

After using a specific guided relaxation procedure in a group session, we solicit feedback from all group members regarding what they experienced during the exercise. This provides an excellent opportunity to identify problems and reinforce approximations of success. An attempt is made to respond positively and with interest to nearly all experiences other than reports of pain. Initially, some patients will report, "it just didn't work" or "I couldn't get into it." In response, the group leader can explore what they had expected to happen and what precisely did occur in their minds during the relaxation exercise. Even reports of pain can sometimes be responded to in a therapeutic way. For example, a patient may state, "I just couldn't relax because my legs were hurting so bad." Our response may then be, "but what about your shoulders and arms, were you able to relax them just a little bit?" In other words, if patients can admit any areas of increased relaxation, we can then respond positively and enthusiastically that they were able to get some relaxing effects in spite of the presence of pain.

Another requirement for relaxation mentioned by Benson (1975) is a passive attitude. It is especially important that patients learn how to manage the inevitable distractions that occur. In fact, the issue of distractions as impediments to time-out relaxation is usually discussed in some detail. Distractions in this context are defined as anything that disrupts sustained focus of attention on the object of relaxation. Distractions can arise from the external environment or from within. External distractions, especially sounds, can be minimized by finding a quiet environment. More problematic are internal distractions that can be either physical or mental. Pain can be a major physical distraction, but it is not necessarily the only one. Relaxation practice can be much more difficult if the person is hungry, thirsty, sexually aroused, or feeling the urge to eliminate. Tight, constrictive clothing can also interfere with relaxation. Most of these physical distractions can be eliminated or minimized through appropriate action. Cognitive distractions can also present problems. Ideally, whenever intrusive thoughts occur, an attempt should be made to return attention back to the object of relaxation. Two extremes should be avoided. First, the person should avoid letting attention be completely carried away by an associative train of distracting thoughts, since the goal of the exercise would then be forgotten. Also to be avoided are attempts to directly force distracting thoughts from awareness. Such attempts are self-defeating and can lead to increased tension. Some patients must be cautioned against trying too hard to achieve particular results. Consequently, patients should be encouraged to attempt to maintain a passive attitude while keeping a concentrative focus on the object of relaxation.

The issue of practice cannot be overemphasized. Patients are asked to practice some form of time-out relaxation at least twice each day. To facilitate practice of relaxation while in the pain program, we use the self-monitoring form shown in Figure 7.1. Patients are instructed to record only those times of practice on their own rather than exercises led by one of their instructors. This form requires patients to record the date,

| Date | Time | Place | Procedure used | Tension level (0–100) | |
				Before	After

FIGURE 7.1.   Relaxation practice monitoring form.

time, place, and type of relaxation exercise. It also asks them to make a subjective estimate of their tension level, using the tension–relaxation continuum described earlier, before and after completing the exercise. These monitoring forms are then reviewed in group sessions. Praise is given to those who report reductions in tension level. Problems encountered during relaxation practice are discussed.

Occasionally, a patient will report an increase in tension after completing a relaxation exercise. In some cases, the patient may be trying too hard to concentrate or produce a desired effect. In other cases, this may be the result of what has been called "relaxation-induced anxiety" (Heide & Borkovec, 1983). If we suspect the latter, we suggest that this is a normal and usually temporary phenomenon, especially for some tense individuals who are just beginning to learn how to relax. The nature of the increased tension should also be determined (e.g., muscle spasms, autonomic arousal, intrusive thoughts and images) and treated accordingly. Sometimes, an alteration in relaxation procedure can be suggested. For example, some patients report increased pain and somatic tension whenever they attempt body-awareness relaxation approaches. Such patients can be encouraged to use external focus or relaxing-imagery approaches.

For other patients, the source of increased anxiety must be addressed more directly. For example, one of our patients reported intrusive images regarding his painful injury nearly every time he closed his eyes to practice a relaxation procedure. Most often he saw images of the individual whom he held responsible for his injury. This resulted in a considerable increase in tension and angry feelings. During a relaxation practice session, another patient experienced a "flash back" to a traumatic childhood sexual experience. Since these patients had previously been attempting to suppress all thoughts associated with their traumatic experiences, attention was given in individual psychotherapy sessions to help them "come to terms" with their traumas.

In addition, many audio cassette relaxation tapes are available including those that are commercially produced as well as those that are designed for patients in a particular program. We have developed a library of about 20 relaxation and pain management tapes in one of the authors' voices that we make available to our patients on a nonprofit basis (i.e., we require that our patients provide the blank cassettes). Patients are cautioned against becoming too dependent on tapes, since they may wish to do time-out relaxation on occasions when a tape or tape player is not available. Tapes can be used to supplement their efforts to practice unaided relaxation techniques.

Relaxation Activities

Relaxation activities occupy an intermediate position between coping relaxation and time-out relaxation. Coping relaxation is used to reduce states of heightened tension. Time-out relaxation is used to bring about deep relaxation. Relaxing activities usually require some degree of concentration and alertness. In addition to serving as methods to counter stress and tension, relaxing activities have other benefits as well. As discussed in Chapter 5, relaxing hobbies and social activities can divert attention away from pain and can serve as the means for deriving positive reinforcement. Patients are encouraged to develop a variety of relaxing activities including those that can be performed alone or with others.

Some physical activities that are not usually considered relaxing can serve an important role in management of excess tension. Especially useful for some individuals are aerobic activities such as jogging or brisk walking, swimming, bicycling, dancing, aerobic exercise classes, etc. Provided the patient does not overtax his or her body, these activities can leave one feeling very relaxed after the activity has been completed.

BIOFEEDBACK, HYPNOSIS, AND SELF-MANAGEMENT

Biofeedback Training

Biofeedback training, including use of electromyographic (EMG) feedback and digital skin temperature feedback, has a varied role in chronic-pain management. With some individuals it may be a very useful treatment modality. For those who present many features of the chronic-pain syndrome, it is rarely effective as a primary treatment approach. Most advocates of biofeedback recommend that it be combined with other approaches (Belar & Kibrick, 1986; Blanchard & Andrasik, 1985). Multi-component chronic-pain management programs vary in their use of biofeedback, with some programs making extensive use of it and others, such as ours, using it infrequently. Research investigations and clinical use of biofeedback training have focused primarily on those with chronic tension or migraine headache (Turner & Chapman, 1982). Biofeedback has also been used for patients with back pain (Belar & Kibrick, 1986). A rationale for the specific use of EMG biofeedback for back pain has been presented by Dolce and Raczynski (1985). Although at one time it was hoped that biofeedback training could directly alter specific physiological mechanisms underlying pain, it is now recognized that most applications of biofeedback training with chronic-pain patients serve to facilitate the acquisition of general relaxation skills.

Rather than relying on biofeedback as a primary relaxation training tool, we have used biofeedback to enhance patients' beliefs in their ability to reduce muscle tension or alter peripheral blood flow through time-out relaxation. Digital or visual displays of EMG or temperature changes can provide patients with concrete evidence that their relaxation exercises are having a beneficial effect on their physiology. In contrast to conventional biofeedback training procedures, we have frequently hooked patients to biofeedback instruments without giving them constant visual or auditory feedback. After a baseline period, they are guided through or instructed to perform on their own a specific relaxation procedure as the therapist monitors changes in the target variable. After completing the relaxation exercise, patients are given feedback regarding the changes that took place as they were becoming progressively relaxed.

When using biofeedback-assisted relaxation, it is also important to emphasize that the specific physiological indices being monitored represent only selected segments of the total relaxation response. Relaxation is a multidimensional process that potentially involves several physiological and cognitive components. Therefore, just because someone does not show significant changes in muscle tension or skin temperature does not necessarily mean that the person is not deriving experiential benefits from a time-out relaxation procedure.

Hypnosis

When one presents various relaxation and imagery procedures, the topic of hypnosis is often raised. Chronic-pain patients' attitudes toward hypnosis vary considerably. Some view it as a potential panacea for their pain, whereas others view it in a much more skeptical light. Although many express some curiosity regarding hypnosis, a few patients are threatened by it and want no part of it. Those who are most negative tend to hold a popular image of the hypnotist as one who is imbued with special power and skill who can exert control over certain people's minds, especially those who are weak, gullible, and highly suggestible. Even less extreme versions of this image run directly counter to the goals of self-management, which emphasize self-control and self-reliance.

Since the term hypnosis so often connotes control by one person (hypnotist) over another, we do not emphasize it in our self-management program. Nevertheless, it is recognized that many of the relaxation and imagery procedures used in our program were derived from practitioners of clinical hypnosis. It is possible to present a standard set of instructions referring to it in one instance as hypnosis and in another as guided imagery or relaxation. Thus, depending on the interest of the group, we may present a pain-modification imagery technique such as glove anesthesia or mobilizing the endorphins (see Chapter 6) as hypnosis or an imagery exercise.

Before labeling a procedure as hypnosis, we discuss the nature of hypnosis in a group session. We begin by defining all hypnosis as self-hypnosis. The point to be made is that for hypnosis to work, the person must participate willingly and actively in the process. No hypnotist can make another person do something that he or she really does not wish to do. We also try to demystify hypnosis by placing it more in the realm of common experience. Following Soskis (1986), we define hypnosis as a process that allows one to experience particular thoughts and images as real. Using this definition, we can point out that common experiences such as becoming absorbed in a good book or an enjoyable movie are forms of self-hypnosis. For example, a person would be unable to enjoy a movie if attention were directed at the reality of the situation (i.e., sitting in a dark theater watching images projected on a two-dimensional screen that consisted of professional actors reciting lines from a script). When attending a movie, people voluntarily agree to suspend "reality" in order to experience as real the events occurring in the movie. As the viewer experiences the movie scenes, he or she may be affected mentally, emotionally, and physiologically. The same process occurs in stage hypnosis that is done for entertainment purposes. Therapeutic self-hypnosis involves experiencing as real particular therapeutic suggestions given by a professional or by the person doing the self-hypnosis.

In the teaching of self-hypnosis, two basic phases are distinguished. First is a process of relaxation and attention narrowing, often referred to as the "induction." In a group setting, patients are taught simple induction procedures such as eye fixation (i.e., staring at a spot on the wall or ceiling until involuntary eye closure is experienced) or arm levitation. If desired, this may be followed by a deepening procedure such as a 10-to-1 countdown accompanied by appropriate imagery (e.g., going down an elevator, escalator, or spiral staircase). Some experience this as a trance state, whereas others prefer to label it as a pleasant state of relaxation. The second stage involves presentation of the therapeutic suggestion, the content of which depends on what the person is trying to accomplish. Suggestions can take the form of verbally stated ideas or images. Suggestions can pertain to the immediate hypnotic experience (e.g., experiencing analgesia in areas of discomfort) or to changes in thinking and behavior following the hypnotic experience. Posthypnotic suggestions can refer to specific changes in habits, modification of dysfunctional attitudes and beliefs, and utilization of more constructive coping behaviors.

To illustrate this process, we guide patients through several examples of hypnotic suggestions centered around self-management themes. One example is modeled after a procedure used in a study by Melzack and Perry (1975, 1980). In this procedure patients are guided through an eye-closure induction and "escalator" countdown followed by a series of "ego-enhancing suggestions." Examples of posthypnotic suggestion themes used in our program include (1) coping with episodes of intense pain, (2) coping with emotional upsets and negative feelings, and (3) self-management of physical activities. Each of these procedures is available on cassette tape. Patients who are interested in this procedure are given encouragement and assistance in developing their own self-hypnosis procedures incorporating personally relevant suggestions. Some record their own suggestions on tape for later playback.

It is far beyond the scope of this book to discuss in detail the clinical use of hypnosis for chronic pain. Most of the approaches have been aimed at modifying the immediate pain experience (e.g., Barber, 1982, 1986; Erickson, 1982; Sacerdote, 1982; Sachs, Feuerstein, & Vitale, 1977). As mentioned above, hypnosis can also be used to reinforce self-management principles and procedures. Thus, our own preference is to present hypnosis as one of many self-management techniques.

SUMMARY

An essential component of self-management training is helping patients cope more effectively with stress and depression. Using a transactional model of pain and stress, self-management training focuses on how the patient cognitively appraises losses and stressful demands, utilizes coping responses, and mobilizes coping resources such as social supports. Patients are first reminded of the various ways that stress, tension, anger, depression, and pain interact. They are then introduced to the basic idea that their perception and interpretation of various events significantly influence their emotional and behavioral responses to such events. Cognitive-therapy procedures are then used to help patients identify and modify some common cognitive distortions that often lead to unnecessary tension, anger, or depression. Cognitive and behavioral coping strategies emphasizing both problem-focused and emotion-focused coping are presented and discussed. The use of general problem-solving skills, assertive communication, constructive actions, and stress-management procedures such as time-out relaxation are reviewed.

CHAPTER 8

The Organization and Management of a Chronic-Pain Program

The efficient organization and administration of a chronic-pain management program (CPMP) are critical to the effectiveness of our treatment model. The most potentially effective clinical interventions will fail if not implemented by a multidisciplinary treatment team that works well together. Additionally, clinic or hospital administrators must work closely and in a supportive manner with CPMP clinical staff to allow treatments to be successfully implemented. Program organization must be clearly delineated yet flexible enough to manage the inevitable unusual, unexpected problems for which no apparent rules exist. In this chapter we describe the organizational structure of a chronic-pain management program based on the self-management model, identify common problems in the administration of such programs, and suggest solutions to these problems. We identify alternative ways to adapt the self-management model to noninstitutional settings.

THE PAIN-CLINIC SETTING

The self-management model would be most effectively implemented within the administrative structure and resources of a multidisciplinary medical center. Yet, because this model deemphasizes traditional medical treatment, the program would ideally be geographically separate from areas that house acutely ill patients. Pain patients are typically ambivalent toward the medical establishment, an attitude that doubtless develops out of a history of dependence on physicians along with a failure to find pain relief through traditional medical intervention. We have found that patients often react poorly to being in an acute-care setting. They are often affected by being near "sick" patients who remind them of their own unsuccessful hospitalizations (see the discussion in Chapter 5 regarding hospital environment cues and their effect on patient behavior). Also we have found that such a setting may have a paradoxical effect on new self-management patients by renewing interest in a medical resolution of their pain (even though they have probably been told there is nothing further medically that can be done for them), which only serves to distract them from attending to the self-management model. Thus, the advantages of being affiliated with such centers are more often practical than therapeutic. For example, physical therapy and other rehabilitation facilities are more readily available in such settings, and thus necessary equipment and staff can be shared with other services. However, the physical separation of the chronic-pain clinic from the hospital is important in reinforcing the idea that the self-management and medical models are distinctly different.

We reinforce the distinction between the pain-program setting and the other hospital sections by implementing certain policies patients must follow. All CPMP patients must wear regular street clothes rather than hospital pajamas. Patients are housed in their own set of rooms in the back of a medical ward. We have arranged to use a separate therapy space that is not used by any other hospital program. This room may be used by the patients instead of the ward dayroom to watch television, talk, or simply for quiet time. Patients are required to make their own beds, clean their own rooms, and eat separately from other patients. They self-administer all nonnarcotic medication just as if they were at home. Thus, patients are rarely on the medical ward except to sleep and bathe. Patients are told from the start that if they become so ill while in the program that they cannot participate in activities, they will be discharged. By treating our program participants as students rather than as typical medical patients, we are communicating the basic self-management premise that they are responsible for themselves not only in their brief time in our program but also in their daily lives outside the hospital.

INPATIENT VERSUS OUTPATIENT

The chronic-pain program ideally should involve a combination of inpatient and outpatient treatment. We have found that the self-management model is best done within a 3- to 4-week inpatient stay. Early control over the treatment environment is critical to later success. We have not found it possible to have most patients withdraw from narcotics on an outpatient basis. Chronic-pain patients become too tempted to use narcotics and other substances when they are not in a therapeutic environment. These patients have also not yet been exposed in any depth to pain-management techniques and thus may see no alternative to taking medication once they are away from the clinic setting. Patients who routinely use narcotics have minimal tolerance for daily pain, as they have typically used such substances whenever they experience discomfort. This p.r.n. ("as needed") self-administration of medication, as pointed out in earlier chapters, may actually serve to increase pain in the long run by developing a destructive cycle of tolerance and dependence. Because patients in the pain program are only beginning to learn alternative ways of coping and are not proficient at this, they may often interfere with their treatment by using narcotics if these drugs are available. The inpatient setting affords control over this situation. We offer narcotics on a time-contingent basis with no p.r.n. usage. Thus, when increased pain is experienced, patients are faced with having to try newly learned self-management techniques and, we hope, experience some degree of success. In the home setting, without the social reinforcement and structure of the clinic, most patients cannot be expected to have such discipline early in their treatment.

There are other practical reasons to set up the CPMP on an inpatient basis. Although some pain programs are exclusively outpatient, perhaps meeting once a week over a period of 2 or 3 months (Turk et al., 1983), we found that intensive indoctrination in the self-management model is critical to program success. Meeting once or twice a week allows too much time between settings for patients to forget information or to be distracted by their many domestic demands. Patients can find multiple reasons to skip a weekly session, arrive late, or schedule alternative activities at the same time as the therapy session. The inpatient approach allows certain patients to be involved in a pain program who otherwise might not to be able to attend on an outpatient basis because they are physically or financially unable to commute. In an inpatient environment, we expect all patients to attend every activity and to be there on time. Patients often think a rigorous full-day schedule will be too demanding, and, given the choice, they may not attend a particular activity, or they may skip an entire day of program activities. Through the encouragement of fellow patients and staff, our patients often find they can do much more than they believed prior to treatment. The following represents a fairly typical inpatient experience:

O.P., a 60-year-old patient with severe degenerative joint disease, although not using narcotics, had been extremely inactive at home and only left his reclining chair a few hours a day. He had almost no social contacts except with his wife, who worked every day. When faced with the 8-hour-day pain program schedule, he became very discouraged and wanted to be discharged immediately after the first day. We let him know that we understood that the first few days of the CPMP are difficult. We encouraged him to take it slowly and do his best but reminded him that he still was required to attend every activity. The other patients encouraged O.P. to participate. They gently teased him, in a way he could accept, about being slow. Their comments would never have been accepted if they had come from a professional staff member. At least one group member kept an informal supervisory watch over O.P. and made sure that he arrived at every activity. Within 2 weeks, O.P. was getting to all activities on time with no assistance. He was successfully functioning on a fairly rigorous 8-hour-a-day schedule.

A patient such as O.P. might well have failed in an outpatient program. The passivity, depression, and low frustration tolerance of many pain patients simply make outpatient treatment too vulnerable to early disillusionment and drop out. Patients learn to appreciate the benefits of the program through their own experience of success. The group inpatient structure makes this success more likely. We have also noticed a significant benefit from open, unscheduled evening hours when patients often discuss their situations with each other. These discussions rarely turn into gripe sessions, especially without staff around to attend to complaints. More often we have observed that these unsupervised groups provide a setting for a relaxed, supportive sharing of experiences and problem solving. We have found it helpful to include these sessions in the written program schedule for 1 hour every evening, calling them "patient review hours." Patients are completely on their own in these meetings and are encouraged to use the time in the most constructive way possible. We are impressed with the results.

The primary disadvantage of inpatient treatment is increased cost for the patient in terms of time and money. Those who are employed may not be able to get sufficient time off from work. The financial costs of 3 to 4 weeks of inpatient treatment, although reasonable when compared to expensive surgical procedures, are prohibitive for most individuals if third-party coverage is not available.

GROUP VERSUS INDIVIDUAL TREATMENT

There are many advantages in providing group over individual treatment within a pain program. First of all, group treatment is a more efficient use of professional resources. Rehabilitation activities such as physical therapy and occupational therapy can be handled on a group basis. Much of the psychological treatment lends itself to a combined lecture/group discussion format. Relaxation techniques and mental-imagery exercises can

be practiced in a group and need not be done on an one-to-one basis. We
have observed the significant value of intragroup reinforcement and support in the success of this approach. Patients often come to our clinic
feeling isolated, depressed, and alone. Their introduction to other individuals who have had similar experiences with chronic pain is usually
very positive, since they suddenly no longer feel alone. They may spend
some time with each other commiserating their various frustrations and
similar domestic concerns.

   Although operant conditioning theory would suggest that such com-
raderie might reinforce pain behavior, we have found that patients, within
the context of a self-management program, quickly extinguish excessive
pain talk. Individuals who exceed a socially acceaptable level in terms of
telling hideous stories about their suffering are usually shunned by fellow
patients, whereas more sociable behavior is rewarded with attention and
support. Pain patients, at least when in the company of their peers as
opposed to staff, do not want to hear about other people's pain for very
long. Instead, they would rather talk about normal life concerns, family
relationships, work, sports, etc. When pain does interfere with more
normal social interaction (e.g., when one patient is in a great deal of pain
and wants to be alone or becomes less talkative), patients are often supportive without being solicitous. They seem to know how to treat each
other without excessive harshness or pity. Thus, the group format takes
on a therapeutic value of great importance.

   One potential difficulty of the group approach should be discussed.
The group cohesiveness that often develops during the course of the
CPMP may sometimes become directed against the program staff. Elsewhere in this book we have discussed the anger many pain patients feel
toward health care personnel. Sometimes this anger can be fueled by the
group. This hostility often takes the form heard in some alcohol treatment
settings: "How can you help us when you aren't an alcoholic?" (substitute
". . . when you don't have a pain problem?"). It reflects suspiciousness of
the helping professional based partly on past disappointing interactions as
well as the more general frustration of continual suffering without apparent hope of relief. Although such comments may be interpreted as a
challenge to the value of the pain program as a whole, they should be
responded to in a nondefensive, supportive way. Patients are expressing
their concern about whether the program staff are actually able to help
them. They may be fearful that this pain program will turn out to be just
one more failure experience. They need reassurance that the program has
been developed out of cumulative experience in treating a large number of
chronic-pain patients. It can be pointed out that the program is also based
on the research findings and clinical experience of many other professionals who have worked with chronic-pain patients. At the same time

we use such comments to clarify our role as teachers, rather than therapists, who are working to help them better manage their own lives with a minimum of dependence on experts. Thus, the chasm between pain patient and health professional, reflected in the differing role of each in the self-management program, can be turned into a therapeutic interaction reinforcing the principles of self-management.

Even if patients truly find that mutual support and group encouragement are the most critical elements of program success, it can still be said that the goal of self-management was reached. In this context, the rapid growth of self-support groups for chronic-pain patients (such as the American Chronic Pain Association) should be strongly encouraged by any professional working with this population. The existence of both formal and informal self-support groups among pain patients is often critical to the long-term success of the self-management model. The inpatient setting allows for a smoother development of such relationships that are particularly important in the beginning stages of self-management training.

THE TREATMENT-RESISTANT PATIENT

Every health care provider is aware that chronic-pain patients have a reputation of being difficult and uncooperative. Even though we attempt to accept into our program only those who initially present themselves as interested and motivated, we sometimes find that patients behave quite differently after being admitted. They may appear minimally interested in learning self-management or overtly disruptive. There are complex psychological explanations why a patient might be uncooperative or even disruptive in the pain program. Of course, it is unrealistic to assume that a chronic-pain patient who has been coping poorly with life would suddenly behave more adaptively when first admitted to a pain program. Most of our patients demonstrate some ambivalence toward full participation in self-management training. Some patients behave in ways that seriously distract other patients from learning. In Chapter 9 we discuss in-depth possible reasons for noncooperation and failure within the pain management program. From a program administrator's point of view, however, these patients must still be managed on a daily basis irrespective of the psychological etiology of their difficult behavior. It is helpful to focus on how best to handle these patients with the least negative effect on the group as a whole.

The most obvious way to minimize the disruptive-patient effect on the CPMP is through identification of such individuals in the preadmission screening (see Chapter 3 for a discussion of the evaluation of pain program candidates). Inappropriate patients should ideally be identified early and referred to a treatment setting more suitable than an inpatient pain program. They might be better managed in a psychiatric outpatient clinic, a drug or alcohol rehabilitation program, or an outpatient pain clinic depending on their particular problems and needs. Once a patient is assessed to be appropriate for intensive inpatient pain-management training, a thorough verbal orientation should be given to all patients that details expectations of their participation in the program. Clarification of these expectations should be made until it is as clear as possible that everyone understands the program structure and functioning. These "rules" are presented in the form of a written contract (see Figure 8.1) that must be signed in order for the patient actually to begin the program.

Certain common problems occur throughout all programs and are usually easy to resolve. For example, patients sometimes are late or absent from activities because of pain. It is immediately made clear to them that this is unacceptable, and, in as supportive a way as possible, they are asked to go to the next activity. Once patients understand that we are asking them to participate as much as they are capable of rather than expecting them to be 100% for the full day, they usually no longer miss activities. Patients also may believe that because they are housed inside a hospital they will be able to have certain medical tests done or perhaps have a medical specialist come by their bed for a consultation. Again, patients are reminded that no medical or surgical care is provided in the program beyond what an emergency might demand. If patients persist in these demands, they are discharged and encouraged to pursue all medical evaluations they believe to be necessary with the understanding that they can contact us at a later date. Another problem behavior that results in discharge from the program is alcohol or illicit drug use during the inpatient stay.

Whereas some of the above examples may not seem too complicated to handle, passive, noncompliant patients present more challenging dilemmas for the program staff. One such patient might spend a considerable amount of time complaining about a particular staff member, scheduling, or even the hospital food. The person often might remark that if all these problems could be solved, much more progress could be made in the program. These criticisms are best responded to in a therapeutic manner. Individuals with these concerns are encouraged to express them directly rather than disrupt the program in a passive–aggressive fashion. Professional staff may serve as models for patients by encouraging frank dialogue about feelings. It is also suggested to these patients that they view imperfections of the CPMP as representative of an imperfect world with which they must cope, rather than wait for things to change to the way they want them to be. We encourage patients to apply the cognitive

The following items are ground rules for participation in our Chronic Pain Management Program. We believe that your agreement to each principle will allow you to achieve maximum benefit from our program.

1. I understand that I will remain in the program for the full 3 weeks only if I am making satisfactory progress in managing my pain. If I am not making satisfactory progress, as judged by the members of the treatment team, I will be discharged earlier.

2. I will complete all assignments as requested by program staff members (e.g., relaxation exercises, pain ratings).

3. I agree to delay all clinic and nonacute medical appointments until after completion of the program unless specifically requested by the Chronic Pain Program medical staff.

4. I will attend all appointments, arriving on time, unless specifically excused by a program staff member.

5. My spouse, or "significant other," will be expected to participate in treatment.

6. I will not use alcohol while in the hospital during the 3 weeks of the program.

7. I agree to the tapering schedule for any narcotic and/or other prescription pain/tranquilizer medication as decided on by the program staff.

8. I agree not to smoke during all group activities.

9. I understand that program staff will in no way involve themselves in the process of any disability claim and/or lawsuit I may have pending.

10. I agree to participate in a follow-up program on discharge, as specified by the program treatment team.

I have read and agree to abide with the above rules of the Chronic Pain Management Program.

Patient Signature   Program Director

_____   _____

FIGURE 8.1. Chronic-Pain Management Program Treatment Contract.

distortion model (see Chapter 7) to coping with aspects of the program they might not agree with. This model suggests that individuals may overfocus on the negative side of events to the exclusion of positive aspects of those same events. Thus, patients who complain unreasonably and excessively about the program are encouraged to consider all they could learn and gain from the program if they would concentrate more on lectures and group discussions. It may also be asked whether these individuals cope with situations outside the hospital with the same critical attitude and whether this has helped them to be happy or to develop social contacts.

At some point it must be decided whether a patient who continues to be disruptive or excessively preoccupied with less relevant aspects of the program should be discharged early. Certainly, individuals who seriously distract other patients from working in the program must be discharged. Usually the remaining patients are appreciative of the staff for sending the patient home. It cannot be overemphasized that patients who are not complying with program demands or making at least minimal progress are best discharged before the end of the program. Their effect on other patients and on staff morale can be very negative. In addition, since self-management training depends on individuals taking responsibility for their lives, patients who do not participate at an acceptable level should experience the consequences by not being allowed to finish the program. Though this may seem to be a harsh attitude, it seems to reflect accurately the contingencies present in the real world to which the patients are preparing to reenter after completing the CPMP.

When patients are asked to leave before completing the program, we make an effort to avoid presenting this decision in a punitive manner. It may suggested that the program is perhaps not what the patient needs at the present time. It should also be noted that in our program, which treats about 100 inpatients per year, only about 8% do not finish the program because of the behaviors described above. Most patients, with the encouragement of their peers and the staff, truly desire to improve and do demonstrate the appropriate amount of effort to profit from self-management training.

THE CPMP DAILY ROUTINE

The daily schedule of program activities must be the result of both practical and clinical considerations. In our inpatient setting, for example, patient activities had to be designed around the times when ward meals were delivered. Staff members' other clinical commitments had to be accommodated. Clinical concerns also were important. Physical therapy seemed best arranged as the first activity of the day. Patients often report significant stiffness and pain on waking. General conditioning exercises aimed at greater flexibility, strength, and mobility help the patient begin the day with more physical stamina. Patients who have experienced benefits from doing early morning exercises are encouraged to continue doing so after the program ends. Our patients eat breakfast after physical therapy, as they understandably prefer not eating just before exercising. The second activity of the day is an avocational workshop program (vocational rehabilitation therapy or VRT) in which individuals learn the value of both distracting activities and socialization in coping with pain. Patients choose from varied options including woodworking, small engine repair, and gardening. They are told that we are not so much interested in their finding a vocational interest in this clinic as we are in their rediscovering the pleasant feeling of being occupied by something they enjoy. In addition, VRT gives staff important information regarding patient standing and sitting tolerance, work habits, and how well the individual is able to appropriately modulate activity levels. As the previous two activities are physically demanding, we have arranged for the third part of the day to be more sedentary.

Self-management training group includes the teaching of relaxation and pain-coping skills, didactic instruction about the nature of chronic pain, and group discussion regarding the relationship between psychological factors and the pain experience. The cognitive therapy group later in the day focuses on a particular aspect of self-management, that of correcting cognitive distortions that create unpleasant emotional experiences for the patient. Also scheduled in the afternoon is another hour of physical exercise, kinesiotherapy (KT), which consists of varied exercise options including swimming, weight training, and exercycling. The emphasis in KT is on upper-body development, muscle strengthening, and increased aerobic capacity. Swimming, in particular, is of great benefit to many pain patients, especially if the pool is heated. We have found that it is the one exercise that almost all pain patients enjoy and plan to continue with after discharge. It is beneficial to schedule swimming later in the day, as it is relaxing and often reduces muscle tension that has built up over the previous hours of activity.

Not all CPMP therapies meet daily. For example, we have found it beneficial to conduct an unstructured group therapy in which patients can discuss any topic just twice per week. This group complements many of the other CPMP therapies that have a didactic/group discussion format. Patients discuss a variety of topics including feelings and attitudes toward the CPMP, relationship difficulties, and vocational concerns. Excessive "pain talk" is discouraged unless it is discussed with an emphasis on problem solving. All patients have individual appointments with a psychologist at least 1 hour per week. In these sessions we conduct our psychosocial history and assessment. Patient participation within the program is discussed with particular emphasis on identifying and working through problems that are impeding the individual's progress in the CPMP. Family members are required to come to at least one of these individual meetings. Individual sessions also can be used to identify significant psychological factors that patients are reluctant to discuss in a group setting. An example follows:

> R.S., a 38-year-old Mexican-American patient, had never spoken to a psychologist prior to coming into the program. He responded slowly but positively to self-management training over the course of the program. In our third individual session, he began to speak about physical and sexual abuse he had suffered as a child from a male relative. Clearly these were powerful emotional events that the patient had never discussed with anyone before. R.S. had suffered severe trauma that had affected him throughout his life, especially in his view of himself as a man. This distorted image aggravated his ability to cope with many life situations, including his chronic pain. The patient was reluctant to discuss these events within the group, although they were clearly relevant to his overall psychological health. Extra individual counseling sessions were scheduled for R.S. During the last week of the program, individual follow-up was arranged. Our work with this patient focused less and less on chronic pain and more on issues of self-esteem and depression.

In this example the individual therapy hour within the generally group-focused program was critical in the identification and eventual resolution of significant psychological factors relevant to the patient's coping ability.

The comprehensive pain program we have tried to design includes important, although brief, contributions from other medical professionals. Registered dieticians provide information about nutrition and weight loss that is important for many of our inactive patients. Individuals benefit greatly from weekly group meetings with successful CPMP graduates who may serve as models for effective coping with pain. These self-support groups often focus on difficulties in interacting with health care professionals and frustrations in applying self-management principles. Our experience with these patient-led groups leads us to believe that they are a necessary aspect of treatment serving a function that cannot be duplicated by a psychologist.

One last aspect of the CPMP schedule should be discussed. We request that patients meet together two evenings per week without professional supervision. These meetings are opportunities for patients to help each other to better understand program content. Often sessions deal with interpersonal problems among patients. Whatever the content of these group meetings, they provide patients with time to discuss application of the self-management model without the added pressure of the "expert" in attendance. Many of our patients tell us that these informal meetings are among the most valuable CPMP experiences.

STAFF ROLES

The effective functioning of a multidisciplinary pain program requires a coordinated, consistent approach by all members of the treatment team. Rather than being a collection of specialists each operating independently, staff members have important responsibilities toward one another. These responsibilities include support of other team members and continuous communication of information about patient progress and program policies. Regular treatment team meetings are essential to this end.

The actual composition of pain-management staff varies from program to program. The minimum staffing requirements for an inpatient self-management pain program should include a physician, adequate nursing staff, a clinical or counseling psychologist, and a physical therapist. Since medical and surgical treatment is de-emphasized in self-management training, the particular physician specialty is less crucial. In our program, physicians are specialists in physiatry (physical medicine). Other members of our treatment team include nursing personnel, clinical psychologists, a social worker, a vocational rehabilitation therapist, a physical therapist, a kinesiotherapist, and a dietician. Brief discussions of the roles of the physician, nurse, psychologist, and physical therapist follow.

Role of the Physician

Since the self-management model encourages the individual to assume the major responsibility for pain control, the traditional role of the physician might seem to be minimal in such a setting. Specific chronic-pain interventions including nerve blocks, neurolytic procedures, electrical-stimulation implants, and other invasive techniques must be done outside of the context of self-management programs. Actually, the role of all health care providers—psychologist, physical therapist, and nurse, for example—could be seen as minimal in a self-management program if approached from a traditional biomedical perspective. As discussed in Chapter 2, this model often requires the patient to play a passive, dependent role, whereas the expert takes an active treatment role. We prefer to view the role of all health care providers from the self-management perspective as being considerably different than in a traditional medical or rehabilitation program.

The physician's role in the pain clinic may have several dimensions. In our program the physician plays a major role in the screening process. The physician makes certain that the prospective patient has been reasonably evaluated medically and that if any medical evaluations or treatments should be completed, they are scheduled as soon as possible. Patients who are no longer appropriate for medical care for their pain problem are the most suitable self-management candidates, and the physician must make this determination prior to psychosocial assessment of the patient. Patients are usually not interested in considering a self-management approach to their pain if they believe that potentially helpful medical procedures are still available. In dealing with this topic, the physician must be able to communicate to the patient in clear terms the reality of his condition and the limits of medicine to deal with it.

Communication skills, then, are particularly relevant to the pain-clinic physician who spends a significant amount of professional time educating patients as opposed to treating them in a traditional "hands on" sense. The physician input once the patient enters the program is also often of a didactic nature. Patients may have questions regarding the medical risk of certain physical exercises they have been asked to do. They have ongoing concerns about their physical condition as the program progresses.

Of course, acute medical problems may arise while the patient is in an inpatient setting. Addressing these medical concerns need not be reinforcing of patients' somatic focus. The physician can take advantage of the patients' concerns by educating them about the use of self-management techniques in coping with pain. As the medical authority on the pain clinic staff, the physician's message to the patient is more critical than that of any other staff member regarding the importance and appropriateness of self-management. The physician who best fits the type of pain program we have been describing is one who achieves professional satisfaction in interactions with patients that are devoid of many of the traditional treatment procedures in which the physician has been trained.

Role of the Nurse

As with the physician, the nurse's role in the CPMP is considerably different from a nurse's traditional responsibilities in an acute-care setting. There is a de-emphasis on the nurse as care giver with an increased role for the nurse as educator or supporter of self-management. The nurse on the hospital ward housing chronic-pain patients is especially important in educating the patient regarding self-management and supporting program goals and therapies. The nurse's reaction to a patient's behavior can be positive (e.g., encouraging of patients to practice self-management procedures, reinforcing indications of progress) or negative (e.g., giving undue attention to pain behavior, expressing anger or disgust at the patient's somatic concerns). As a member of the identified medical staff (as compared to the nonmedical professional staff of psychologists, social workers, etc.), the nurse's strong endorsement of self-management has an especially positive impact on patient attitudes.

Copp (1987) writes about common biases regarding patients in pain that nurses (and others) hold that may interfere with successful pain management. One of these biases is seen in the statement "patients cannot be trusted to take their own medication." We have seen this bias operate in our program, where a nurse expressed great distrust that a patient could take appropriate levels of his prescribed medication. Of course, the patient had been fully responsible for taking his own medication prior to his admission to the program and would be equally responsible after discharge. He felt that such distrust was unwarranted and contraindicated the goals of the program. Here the two basic models of pain treatment clashed. The traditional approach assumes that hospitalized patients are too ill to manage their own medications. In a self-management program, patients are continually faced with the realization that they are responsible for dealing with their condition. In the above case, the nurse's concern over the patient's medication could have been approached from the self-management perspective by emphasizing education and instructing the patient to take medication appropriately.

Role of the Psychologist

Throughout this book we have discussed psychological assessment and intervention strategies that the CPMP psychologist would most likely be responsible for implementing. In addition to these direct clinical services, most psychologists have been trained to conduct research and program evaluation studies. At the very least, each pain program should have a built-in program evaluation component that can enable staff to assess program efficacy.

The psychologist may also be an appropriate choice for sharing administrative responsibilities. In hospital-based programs, it is not uncommon for the psychologist to serve as codirector along with a physician. In self-management pain programs, administration centers around the successful implementation of behavior-change principles. The program director's psychological expertise may be used to negotiate patient–staff or intrastaff conflicts, resolve incidents of patient noncompliance, and make numerous program policy decisions regarding patient management. Thus, the psychologist may contribute in four distinct ways to the CPMP: (1) administration and program management, (2) research and program evaluation, (3) patient assessment, and (4) treatment.

Role of the Physical Therapist

The physical therapist has always played an integral role in the chronic-pain program (Doliber, 1984). As part of the treatment team, the physical therapist is involved in developing group exercise programs, providing instruction in proper body mechanics, and supervising TENS usage. Individualized exercise instruction is also part of the physical therapist's input. We concur with the often expressed belief that the physical therapist should emphasize active coping approaches as opposed to passive procedures such as various types of massage and ultrasound. In keeping with our basic paradigm, all methods that increase an individual's ability to cope with his or her pain without depending on others are encouraged.

Thus, although TENS involves an instrument that does something to the patient, it is controlled by the patient in terms of when and how it is used. More passive modalities could easily encourage patients to depend on family members or professionals to deliver the treatment. This dependence adds to the patient's sense of diminished control and can further the depressive spiral. The benefit of minimal, and often temporary, pain relief from passive treatment modalities may be outweighed by the negative psychological effects of using a technique that maintains or even increases dependence on others. The physical therapist's role in teaching and encouraging patients to take control of their physical exercise regimens is critical to the successful implementation of the self-management model.

Most chronic-pain patients believe that they have been told by their physician to minimize physical activity as a way to minimize pain. Past exercise programs have usually failed, as the patient has either done exercises incorrectly or has had unrealistic expectations of what daily exercise could accomplish (i.e., "it would help take my pain away"). The encouragement of daily exercise allows the patient to feel an increasing sense of well-being and self-control. Such exercise regimens strengthen muscles, increase mobility and flexibility, and stimulate local circulation (Clelland, Savinar, & Shepard, 1987).

The pain program physical therapist may face numerous sources of patient resistance. Patients are often reluctant to try a particular exercise because they have been told that it may aggravate their condition. The physical therapist often judges that the exercise would be of benefit. In this example, the physical therapist's understanding of the difference between acute and chronic pain is most important. The patient must realize that in the acute-pain phase, often after a traumatic injury, exercise is inappropriate, as injured tissue needs time to repair itself. If such inactivity is continued, however, the patient puts him- or herself at greater risk for increased pain because of poor flexibility and mobility as well as increased depression. If the patient operates from the biomedical model, the physical therapist's instructions will seem unsatisfactory and countertherapeutic. The patient may better understand the importance of regular exercise as he is exposed to the principles of self-management in the other phases of the entire treatment program.

Exercises that seem to increase pain often cause patients to stop exercising altogether. The physical therapist may suggest modification of exercises and utilize the principles discussed in Chapter 4. Patients must understand that not all pain they experience during and after exercise is caused by their chronic-pain condition but may be the result of a positive attempt to become physically stronger. The pain patient group members may exert significant influence over each other in helping to understand and accept the physical therapists' exercise prescriptions and ideas regarding the importance of exercise. The physical therapists in our program support this group cohesiveness by having patients do certain exercises together and having participants take turns leading the rest of the group through a particular exercise sequence. The self-management perspective requires the patient to be responsible for completing his or her exercises, with the physical therapist acting more as a coach who offers guidance and encouragement. Such an approach better prepares the individual for implementing an appropriate post-hospital exercise program based on what had been learned in physical therapy.

THE CPMP AS A TRAINING EXPERIENCE

Pain programs that are based in teaching hospitals may serve an useful function in the training of health care professionals. Predoctoral psychology interns play an important role in our program. Working with the chronic-pain patient allows the intern considerable exposure to the effects of chronic illness on individuals and their families. Experience in consulting with other staff is also readily available. Interns value the opportunity to learn the therapeutic techniques we use, many of which are applicable to a wide variety of nonpain patients. Interns have first-hand exposure to the influence of large institutional systems such as medical facilities and compensation and disability regulators on an individual's attempts to cope with illness and disability.

Medical residents also are part of our CPMP staff. Because pain is the major symptom that motivates most individuals to go to a physician, the broader biopsychosocial perspective on pain emphasized in the pain program better prepares the physician-in-training for future patient contacts. Residents have the opportunity to work with chronically ill patients who are best helped by nontraditional interventions. The recognition of the limitations of traditional medical techniques may be a valuable aspect of the resident's work with the chronic-pain patient. As we indicated above when discussing the role of the physician in the CPMP, the pain-program setting demands on the physician include critical skills such as patient education, communication of concern and reassurance to anxious or angry individuals, and physical assessment. All of these opportunities are of clear benefit to the resident's training irrespective of the subspecialty of medicine he or she eventually chooses.

Although we have had little experience with students from other disciplines, the CPMP would seem to provide relevant training opportunities for any future health care professional, since pain is a primary focus of many different types of patients. The exposure to an alternative model of pain and illness behavior could only better prepare students for their interactions with the complex realities of care of chronically ill patients.

ALTERNATIVES TO COMPREHENSIVE INPATIENT PAIN PROGRAMS

The intensive inpatient pain program we have been describing throughout the preceding pages is not practical for all settings. The basic self-management philosophy, however, is applicable, with modification, in any professional interaction with the chronic-pain patient. In this section we discuss how to adapt the treatment model to outpatient settings.

Many pain clinics follow the basic tenets of the self-management model on an outpatient basis. Outpatient pain programs may be set up in a number of alternative ways depending on the particular treatment and staffing possibilities available at a clinical facility. One type of program could be designed on a day hospital basis with patients attending for full 8-hour days, 5 days a week. Other options could include fewer full or half-day programs. We are familiar with many outpatient pain programs representing a variety of lengths and designs.

The self-management approach can be adapted to any type of treatment setting, whether outpatient or inpatient, and irrespective of possible program length. We believe, however, that outpatient pain management success depends on strongly motivated patients who can function at a significant level of independence prior to beginning treatment. The most challenging of the chronic-pain patients may have difficulty complying with the full-day pain program on an outpatient basis. Such patients often find it troublesome to come to the clinic regularly because of early morning pain that is commonly found in chronic patients. Clinic times could be arranged with consideration of these factors, with later starting times or half-day programs. Narcotic reduction, then, would be essentially self-managed by the patient. This can often be very difficult for the patient new to the nonmedical coping approach. Staff can help develop a tapering schedule and monitor compliance with the schedule through self-report. The accuracy of this method is limited by patient honesty. Patients can be encouraged in their attempt to reduce the use of narcotics, and problems with reduction can be addressed and resolved in clinic meetings.

Although the inpatient setting allows controlled distribution of medications that is an advantage early in treatment, the outpatient setting provides a more realistic opportunity for the patient to generalize treatment effects from the clinic to the home environment. Patients who are more narcotic-dependent and express less enthusiasm for the self-management approach and those who have little positive social support at home usually find narcotic reduction on an outpatient basis to be much more difficult. These individuals may better be served in an inpatient setting whenever possible.

The outpatient clinic can present all of the relevant psychological and physical self-management principles and techniques in as much depth as is done within the inpatient format. Significant differences between the two program arrangements have much to do with how well the patient is able to focus on the therapeutic material concurrently with facing the demands of their often stressful home environment on a daily basis. Although home stresses and their management are, of course, a major topic within the inpatient group, they may present more immediate problems for the outpatient pain patient who knows he must deal with the problems each evening after attending the pain clinic. Ongoing home stresses can be addressed on a daily basis from within the self-management framework to allow the patient to see the immediate application of the principles to improved coping. If these real-life concerns are partially ignored and too much emphasis is placed on didactic instruction or the following of a set therapeutic agenda, some patients may become distracted by external stresses and find it very difficult to participate in the pain clinic. The inpatient setting may afford some necessary respite from these problems while helping to prepare the patient for coping more successfully on discharge. Of course, outpatient treatment may be advantageous in that relevant life stresses can be monitored on a daily basis and patients have an immediate opportunity to apply newly learned coping skills. This can result in greater generalization of treatment effects. Ideally, we would design a program that begins with an intensive introduction in self-management on a group inpatient basis followed by intermittent but long-term group or individual outpatient sessions that offer ongoing reinforcement of coping principles.

PROGRAM FOLLOW-UP

Periodic therapeutic follow-up is an important aspect of the self-management model. This suggestion may seem to contradict the model's emphasis on individual responsibility for coping with pain without dependence on health care professionals. However, it is unrealistic to expect most patients to be able to manage their pain effectively after participating in a relatively brief inpatient or outpatient pain program without occasional professional support. The format of this assistance should be designed to maximize independent coping skills. Our weekly follow-up support group is available to all inpatient program graduates. Problem solving, ventilation of feelings, practicing stress-reducing mental exercises, and identifying ways of coping with severe pain episodes are common topics in the group.

Patients are encouraged to bring spouses and other family and friends to the group so that they can also participate in discussions. This group is designed on an open basis with all appropriate patients welcome each session without an appointment. An open format increases patient attendance by eliminating any bureaucratic hurdles to participation. Usually a core group of patients and spouses attend frequently, with another set of patients participating on a regular but infrequent basis. Patients who are months or years post-treatment can offer significant assistance to recently discharged individuals. Group sessions may have set agendas in which the psychologist initiates discussion around a particular topic or shares information about pain management gathered from recent publications or professional meetings. Other group sessions are unstructured and focus on whatever themes patients identify as a priority that week.

In addition to this open follow-up support group, we have developed a couples group for those whose pain has significantly impacted on the marital relationship. In some cases both spouses have a chronic-pain condition. This group is also held on a weekly basis and is limited to five or six invited couples. Group participants are responsible for initiating discussion, with group leaders serving as facilitators.

Individual follow-up sessions can be important for certain patients, although they are time consuming and costly from a professional's point of view. We encourage group sessions in most cases not only because they are more cost-effective but also because of the positive influence of the group on patients' coping abilities. Individualized meetings are necessary when patients express general discomfort with group participation or need to address specific subjects that they are uncomfortable discussing in front of other people. More "personal" topics such as sexual problems, alcohol or drug use, or severe marital discord may be subjects that some patients would feel more comfortable discussing within an individual therapy format. Very often patients in the pain program will identify psychosocial problems that they were previously unaware of or unwilling to address until placed in a therapeutic environment. Many times these problems reflect serious long-term difficulties that could not possibly be resolved within the short time the patients are in the pain program. Examples include the effects of childhood physical and sexual abuse, long-term passive personality disorder, serious long-term substance abuse, and varied childhood-related psychological conflicts. As will be discussed in Chapter 9, these problems often require more extensive psychotherapeutic approaches.

It is revealing about the nature of chronic-pain patients that given the opportunity to talk about difficult subjects other than pain, patients often are willing to discuss matters of great psychological concern within a relatively short period of time. These difficult issues have been buried by the patients as they have focused on their physical discomfort. It is only within a psychologically oriented pain program that such issues are exposed, since the majority of our patients have had minimal or no prior therapeutic contact with a mental health professional. Following up on these serious psychosocial matters is a critical part of the comprehensive pain program and seems to help strengthen a patient's ability to cope effectively with his or her present life including pain-related stressors. Many of these more sensitive concerns need to be addressed on an individual basis, but even when individual counseling is the preferred approach, the patients may still be encouraged concurrently to attend the follow-up support group.

In our program, many patients do not live close enough to the treatment facility to attend postprogram outpatient groups. Other pain clinics may have similar obstacles to having certain patients return for follow-up, such as transportation limitations, work schedules, and financial considerations. Alternative follow-up arrangements should be developed. Some of our pain program graduates have organized their own support groups in their local communities.

Written materials describing program content can be taken home by patients, who can then refer to self-management concepts as needed in the home environment. Each patient attending our inpatient program receives a spiral notebook containing handouts of self-management topics. Appropriate articles and books written for lay people may also be suggested. We provide patients with a reading list of books that amplify various self-management themes. Of the many popular books written for chronic-pain patients, we particularly recommend Sternbach's (1987) book entitled *Mastering Pain: A Twelve-Step Program for Coping with Chronic Pain*, which is currently available in paperback. As mentioned earlier, patients also leave our program with relaxation tapes that they are encouraged to use whenever needed.

Phone accessibility is critical for successful follow-up. Patients need to know that therapists are, within reason, available to them for support and clarification about pain-management techniques. We make a concerted effort to identify qualified professionals in the area in which the patient lives to refer program graduates for community follow-up. We have found it beneficial to send program information to these therapists and to have telephone contact with them whenever possible. Sometimes we have found it necessary to readmit individuals to the inpatient program if outpatient follow-up is simply not working.

T.U. was a 47-year-old patient with low back pain for 20 years. He did well in our program, but on returning to his home 1,000 miles from our facility, he faced new family and financial demands that could not have been anticipated when he was in the program. He faced these new stressors, although there was little available professional support to reinforce self-management principles. When our telephone contacts with T.U. did not seem to be helping any longer, he asked to return for a refresher course. He had benefited from his previous experience at our clinic, so we decided to approve his request to be readmitted. He did well on his repeat visit and returned home better prepared to manage his many domestic problems.

It is not realistic to think that every patient will profit equally from the inpatient program. We have been impressed by how certain individuals do not seem to grasp self-management principles until late in the program, but when these same patients are seen for a repeat program, they advance quickly and make great progress. Although it is clearly more difficult to provide adequate postprogram care for individuals who are unable to attend follow-up sessions, adjustments in treatment routine such as those described above can be made in order to maximize generalization of program effect to the home.

EVALUATION OF PROGRAM EFFICACY

Pain programs, irrespective of treatment format and structure, have a responsibility to evaluate their effectiveness. Comparative research studies that have attempted to identify programmatic factors that lead to greater effectiveness in pain treatment have been minimally successful (Turner & Chapman, 1982). Studies are difficult to compare because of varied patient groups in which populations differ widely on relevant demographic criteria (Holzman et al., 1985). Treatment may be evaluated by differing psychological measures that have varying degrees of reliability and validity. There is also a lack of clarity regarding the specific attributes of treatment approaches. For example, "cognitive–behavioral" and "relaxation training" as descriptors of treatment techniques do not allow appropriate comparison across programs because of the different ways such techniques may be designed and implemented. Research on program effectiveness also lacks well-identified control group comparisons, making the comparison of different therapy formats difficult. Thus, evaluation studies have yet to answer the fundamental question of which types of patients are best treated in which kinds of programs. Whereas true controlled studies of pain program effectiveness are difficult to conduct, there is a developing body of data that indicates with some consistency the general value of multidisciplinary, psychologically focused pain programs (Aronoff & Wagner, 1987).

The many complications of program evaluation should not, however, prevent each pain clinic from making a reasonable attempt to measure the impact of its interventions. Ongoing evaluation should lead to modification of treatment approaches and, when indicated, the revamping of program structure. Such positive changes will be reflected in greater patient satisfaction and positive feedback from referral sources. At this stage of our understanding of how best to treat chronic-pain patients, it seems improbable that we will identify one variable that alone measures treatment success. Multidimensional evaluation incorporating many different outcome factors is the preferred method.

In Williams' (1988) review of multidisciplinary pain program evaluation measures, six categories of potential outcome variables are suggested. Physical measures may include self-reports of pain and other physical symptoms, EMG activity, pressure algometry (for trigger and tender points), range of motion, muscle strength, and aerobic fitness. Functional measures may assess disability behavior, productivity, and self-care activity. Behavioral–cognitive variables may include degree of somatic concern, medical utilization, drug usage, verbal and nonverbal pain behavior, sleep disturbance, pain-coping strategies, and self-efficacy measures. Emotional factors can be assessed using various self-report measures of depression and anxiety. Economic factors such as the costs of treatment and disability compensation should also be considered. Finally, a variety of sociocultural factors may be assessed, including living situation, litigation, family involvement, quality of life, and patient goals. Most of these variables can be assessed through patient self-report, questionnaires, or reports from family members. Some of the physical measures require special testing procedures.

Typically, assessment of patient response to treatment begins with use of pre- and posttreatment measures. Many of the variables listed above can easily be assessed at the beginning and immediately after treatment. These include physical, functional, cognitive–behavioral, and emotional measures. In addition to assessing patients' immediate responses to treatment, we believe it is important to elicit patient feedback regarding the program itself. Consequently, we require patients to fill out a questionnaire that asks them to rate the degree of perceived benefit from each of our program components. We also solicit responses to open-ended questions regarding what they found especially helpful or unhelpful, suggestions for improvement, and other comments regarding the program.

Although pre–post program evaluation is necessary, it has been frequently pointed out that the most significant indicator of pain program success is maintenance of benefits months and years after treatment. Research studies have assessed continued patient improvement, usually at 6 months and 1 year post-treatment (Tan, 1982). Ideally this follow-up evaluation should be done within an interview format in the hope of making the contact as therapeutic as possible. Questionnaires are a reasonable alternative, although return rates with such an approach are often disappointing. At the follow-up evaluation, other relevant outcome factors should be assessed. These include longer-term analgesic use, utilization of medical facilities for pain-related problems, vocational status, economic and sociocultural factors, as well as other psychological and physical factors previously assessed at the beginning and end of the program.

SUMMARY

The success of the self-management program approach to chronic pain depends on the appropriate organization of the multidisciplinary program. Professional roles in the program will be somewhat different from those found in acute-care settings. The inpatient pain program offers significant advantages for the patient, as does a group treatment focus. Alternative settings and organization for pain clinics, depending on financial and institutional resources, are discussed in this chapter. Outpatient follow-up of patients is critical to the maintenance of treatment effect. No matter what setting the pain program is in, passively resistant and openly disruptive pain patients present management problems that must be addressed effectively. Proper psychological assessment as well as program evaluation are important considerations in the design of the pain management program. Finally, the staff expectations of the patients participating in the chronic-pain management program must be discussed openly and agreed to by all program participants.

CHAPTER 9

Beyond Self-Management Training

Throughout this book we have presented our views regarding the major factors that contribute to the maintenance of chronic pain. We have further asserted our belief that a comprehensive self-management program is the most efficacious treatment approach. In this chapter, we qualify this belief by discussing patients who are not well suited for self-management training even though it is apparent that psychosocial factors play a significant contributing role to their pain. It must be recognized that, in spite of our best efforts, some chronic-pain patients fail to respond to treatment. Of course the same can be said for attempts to treat any number of conditions. It is often tempting to blame the patient for treatment failure. We can say that the patient was "resistant," "poorly motivated," "uncooperative," or "noncompliant." Although this view reduces our own responsibility, it is not a very satisfying answer. Consequently, much has been written about ways to reduce resistance and increase motivation, cooperation, and adherence to treatment programs (e.g., DiMatteo & DiNicola, 1982; Gerber & Nehemkis, 1986; Meichenbaum & Turk, 1987; Wachtel, 1982). Although failure to cooperate and adhere to treatment programs is a significant reason for unsuccessful outcomes, it is not the only reason. Some patients do cooperate with pain treatments and follow the expert's recommendations but still fail to get better.

One important issue we should like to address in this chapter is problem identification. Complaints of pain and associated pain and disability behavior can occur for a wide variety of reasons. A biopsychosocial systems model of pain, in contrast to the biomedical model, allows for several interacting factors that might serve as causal variables including physiological, emotional, cognitive, behavioral, and environmental factors. We believe that pain treatments sometimes do not succeed because health care practitioners fail to identify correctly the most important factors responsible for maintaining a patient's pain. Furthermore, practitioners often fail to recognize that their professional training and particular specialty can result in considerable bias regarding the specific types of causal factors they consider. This bias then extends to their choice of treatment strategies.

We believe that a cognitive–behavioral treatment model that incorporates physical reconditioning approaches has the most to offer for the greatest number of chronic-pain patients. However, as mentioned at the beginning of Chapter 3, this approach is required only for those who present the chronic-pain syndrome. Although this constitutes the majority of patients who are referred to us (and to other specialty pain clinics as well), it does not necessarily represent the entire population of individuals with a chronic-pain condition.

Those individuals who present many features of the chronic-pain syndrome, such as narcotic dependence, pain preoccupation, depression, social withdrawal, and excessive disability behavior, usually require psychologically based treatment approaches. Nevertheless, it is important to recognize some of the underlying assumptions and limitations inherent in the self-management treatment approach. A major assumption underlying our program and related programs is that patients present either deficits in pain-coping skills (Turk et al., 1983) or excessive reinforcement for maladaptive chronic-pain behavior (Fordyce, 1976). Consequently, it is assumed that a combination of instructional strategies and enhanced incentives for change will result in effective self-management of pain. Specific instructional strategies include lecture, discussion, skills training and rehearsal, modeling, positive reinforcement, and performance feedback. Incentives for change are facilitated through manipulation of environmental reinforcement contingencies and development of a collaborative therapeutic relationship.

Unfortunately, some patients fail to respond to this treatment approach. Following intensive self-management training, they may revert back to excessive pain preoccupation, inactivity, abuse of pain medication, or demands on medical care providers to "do something" to alleviate their pain. In such cases, failure is often attributed to noncompliance with treatment (e.g., continued use of relaxation techniques, maintaining a physical exercise regimen) or inability to modify major environmental reinforcement systems such as disability compensation, pathological family systems, or physicians who encourage a continued search for medical/surgical solutions.

Based on clinical experience, we would suggest that treatment failures are more likely to occur when pain is not the primary problem but instead is symptomatic of some other more fundamental psychological problem. In such cases, the patient may be in need of more traditional psychotherapeutic approaches rather than self-management training and physical reconditioning. Thus, intensive training in pain-coping skills or manipulation of environmental reinforcers for pain behavior during a period of hospitalization may not be the most appropriate treatment. Additional medical/surgical treatment is even more inappropriate with such patients. When self-management approaches fail, the patient is generally not harmed. This is not always the case, however, for pharmacological or surgical pain-control techniques.

We now discuss some examples of patients for whom pain does not appear to be the primary problem. At least four general categories can be distinguished. First, there are those cases in which the presentation of chronic somatic pain may be regarded as a more socially acceptable means of seeking help for current psychosocial problems. Second, we see cases in which the chronic-pain syndrome appears to reflect earlier emotionally painful experiences. In the third category, the presentation of a chronic-pain syndrome may be viewed primarily as a partial solution to other more fundamental psychological problems. Finally, there are those patients whose pain serves to stabilize a family or marital system. Although these four categories are by no means mutually exclusive, we consider them separately.

PAIN AS A MEANS OF SEEKING HELP

Some patients present pain complaints or other somatic symptoms as a means of expressing or seeking help for psychosocial problems. This is not to suggest that they are consciously fabricating somatic complaints. They may be selectively focusing on the somatic correlates of emotional problems. Instead of consciously identifying and seeking help for the real problem, they consult medical practitioners regarding the somatic problem. The following case is an example:

W.Y., a 73-year-old male patient, was referred following repeated visits for recurrent headaches. The patient's symptoms were consistent with a diagnosis of tension headache. During the pain-screening interview, it became apparent that W.Y. had become depressed and lonely following the death of his wife approximately 1 year earlier. He felt alienated from his children and had no close social ties. It was then hypothesized that his recurrent headaches and repeat visits to the outpatient clinic were a result of these psychosocial issues. Rather than offer him training in headache management, we referred W.Y. to a group comprised of patients with similar somatic complaints. This group helped him address his real concerns such as coping with grief and loneliness. When he was able to reestablish social ties and resume solitary activities that had previously given him enjoyment (e.g., writing stories, painting, and photography), his head-ache complaints ceased.

As this case illustrates, pain management was not the patient's major problem even though it was the basis for his seeking professional help. During his entire adult life, W.Y. had prided himself on his emotional fortitude and independence even though he probably had been dependent on his wife for both emotional support and arrangement of social activity. Thus, it was difficult for him to request help for his real problem, as this would have been contrary to his self-image. Once he was encouraged to address the real issues, pain was no longer a focus of concern.

The following is a more complicated case in which pain complaints were used to seek help for other problems.

> A.C. was a 59-year-old divorced woman who presented complaints of chronic abdominal pain. She had a history of peptic ulcer disease and had undergone surgery for this problem several years previously. Since she had not responded to medical treatment, she was referred for pain-management training. Our initial evaluation indicated an anxious, mildly depressed woman who had a number of worries and concerns apart from her physical health. Rather than admitting her to the pain program, we referred her for individual psychotherapy. During the course of therapy, A.C.'s real issues were gradually identified and addressed. These included unresolved anger at her ex-husband for leaving her for a younger woman, concerns about growing old and losing physical attractiveness, excessive dependency on a son who was planning to move out of the area, and a lack of assertiveness. After a few months she was also able to admit to her therapist that she had been secretly abusing alcohol for several years and had hidden this fact from her physicians. It then became apparent that excessive alcohol use was an important factor contributing to her chronic abdominal pain. After undergoing treatment in an alcohol program, her physical problems improved considerably.

In both of these cases, it was readily apparent from the initial evalua-tion that coping with pain was not the primary problem, even though it had been the basis for referral. It took relatively little effort to get these patients to recognize and talk about their real concerns even though neither had ever sought professional help for a psychological problem. Once they were given permission and encouraged to address their psy-chosocial problems, pain quickly became a secondary issue. Individuals such as these do not require a chronic-pain management program. Instead they need individual or group counseling. If the focus of inquiry had been limited to their pain problem and other psychosocial factors had been ignored, they might have been admitted to a structured pain program. In the pain-clinic setting, it is possible that their real problems might have been overlooked or at least not adequately addressed. Unfortunately, it is not always easy to determine from an initial evaluation whether coping with pain, as opposed to some other psychological problem, should be the primary focus with a particular patient.

Some patients initially present themselves as suffering primarily from chronic pain and de-emphasize or even deny other areas of concern. An example of this is the following case:

> B.D. was a 43-year-old married woman with a 12-year history of intermittent low back pain. During the previous year, her pain had reportedly increased in severity. Medical evaluation indicated that she was not a surgical candidate. After failing to respond to a course of physical therapy, B.D. was considered an appropriate candidate for our pain-management program. Although initially she focused on her pain, she gradually began to disclose significant worries regarding her husband whom she suspected was having an extramarital affair. Even though she had never discussed the matter with him, she had significant fears that he might leave her. On confronting him in the presence of her pain-program counselor, she discovered that her husband had indeed been engaging in an affair. At the same time, he insisted that he did not wish to end the marriage. Following this session, the couple was seen for marital counseling.

Although this woman's pain complaints were real enough, pain was not her primary problem. Since she had already learned over the years how to cope with back pain, she did not really need intensive training in pain management. Once she was able to acknowledge her real concerns and participate in marital counseling, back pain was no longer an issue for this patient.

Thus, some people present legitimate complaints of pain even though pain management is not their primary problem. These complaints are symptomatic of other psychosocial problems that result in depression, loneliness, anxiety, and fear. Rather than admit these problems and seek psychological counseling, patients may seek medical assistance for pain. In some cases, the onset of pain complaints coincides with the occurrence of psychosocial problems. In other cases, a preexisting chronic-pain condition becomes exacerbated as a result of psychosocial problems. In either case, these patients usually do not require a comprehensive chronic-pain management program, since once their real concerns are addressed, pain is no longer the primary basis of distress.

PAIN AS A REFLECTION
OF EARLIER LIFE EVENTS

As suggested by pain specialists with a psychodynamic orientation, chronic pain can sometimes reflect traumatic events experienced earlier in life. This can occur when the painful emotional concomitants of these experiences are inhibited and repressed. Depression and substance abuse are commonly found before onset of the pain problem. Typically, the chronic-pain syndrome begins with an actual physical injury, which in some cases may be relatively minor. Pain persists, however, long after the physical injury has healed. The following two cases are examples:

> C.E. was a 34-year-old male who had a 12-year history of chronic low back and right leg pain following a minor back injury. Lumbar disk surgery not only failed to alleviate pain but reportedly increased it. When he was admitted to our program, he was unemployed, narcotic-dependent, moderately depressed, and preoccupied with multiple somatic complaints. During the course of individual counseling, it was discovered that when C.E. was 10 years old his mother had died of a stroke after spending 18 months in a coma. During the months prior to her death, he had accompanied his father to visit her every night in the hospital. These events were reported in a matter-of-fact manner with little affect. When asked how he felt about this unfortunate event, C.E. stated that he could not remember feeling anything and that at no time had he shed tears. When asked why, he stated, "we just didn't show emotion in my family." The patient also admitted that following his mother's stroke, his father began to drink heavily.

The second case illustrates earlier painful experiences and resulting emotional conflict:

> D.F. was a 57-year-old divorced woman who had complained of chronic neck pain for 5 years. No clear medical findings were apparent other than osteoarthritis. She had also had a history of depression and substance abuse prior to development of her pain condition. Although she showed some benefit from the pain-management program, D.F. continued to be depressed in spite of treatment with several antidepressants. Consequently, she was seen for individual psychotherapy. Although we initially utilized a present-focused cognitive therapy approach as discussed in Chapter 7, we eventually considered it important to focus on developmental antecedents. It was discovered that during her first 6 years of life, D.F.'s mother had suffered from tuberculosis and had been confined to a sanitorium for lengthy periods of time. Around age 4, her younger sister died. D.F. remembered her father as being a rather stoical man who stopped

paying much attention to her after the sister died. It was hypothesized that infantile feelings of rage resulting from maternal abandonment had to be repressed because the mother was obviously ill; and that when she was home, everyone had to avoid upsetting her in any way. The patient also experienced guilt that perhaps it was her fault that mother had to go away or that her sister had died. As a consequence, this patient later developed a pattern of polysubstance abuse, self-injurious behavior, unsuccessful intimate relationships, depression, and chronic pain.

In addition to death or separation from a parent, we have encountered cases where earlier life traumas involved significant physical or sexual abuse, emotional neglect, or inconsistent care-giving from parents who appeared to be emotionally disturbed or chemically dependent (most often alcoholic). The occurrence of significant problems during childhood among those with chronic pain has been noted by several others as well (e.g., Adler, Zlot, Hurny, & Minder, 1989; Blumer & Heilbronn, 1982; Engel, 1959; Violon, 1982).

Another type of traumatic experience that we have encountered in our work with veterans concerns war-related experiences. For example, we have treated former prisoners of war as well as those who suffered other traumatic experiences while serving in Viet Nam. Some of these individuals met the diagnostic criteria for posttraumatic stress disorder. It is significant that such traumatic experiences occurred prior to the development of their chronic-pain syndrome.

This is not to suggest that these earlier experiences had directly caused the chronic-pain syndrome. Certainly many individuals suffer such experiences without ever developing chronic pain. Typically, patients not only deny the relevance of these events to their pain but also tend to disclose such experiences reluctantly. Consequently, the assertion that earlier events contribute to the etiology of chronic pain has been based primarily on clinical observation and inference. From our perspective, such observations best fit a general diathesis–stress model. In this case, certain childhood experiences or other traumatic life events may predispose the individual to develop a chronic-pain syndrome if those experiences are not adequately resolved, processed, or integrated on an emotional level. Thus, according to one psychoanalytic writer, "it is not the trauma itself that is the source of illness but the unconscious, repressed, hopeless despair over not being allowed to give expression to what one has suffered and the fact that one is not allowed to show and unable to experience feelings of rage, anger, humiliation, despair, helplessness, and sadness" (Miller, 1984, p.259). As a result, these individuals can develop significant deficits in their "sense of self." In Engel's (1959) term, they become "pain-prone." Later, stressful life experiences, including painful injuries and diseases, can then initiate the chronic-pain syndrome.

Depression as a Mediating Link

The most frequently mentioned mediating link between earlier experiences and chronic pain is depression (e.g., Beutler, Engel, Oro'-Beutler, Daldrup, & Meredith, 1986; Romano & Turner, 1985; Violon, 1982). Although the relationship between chronic pain and depression is complex and variable, the general assumption made by some psychodynamic theorists is that problems in early development result in certain personality traits and depressive tendencies that facilitate the development of chronic pain. For example, Blumer and Heilbronn (1982) suggest that all chronic pain of uncertain etiology is a variant of depression. It is hypothesized that pain patients develop a form of "masked depression," since they are unable to recognize and verbalize their real feelings. As a result of this tendency, referred to as "alexithymia" (Sifneos, 1973), patients express their emotional pain (i.e., depression) in the form of somatic pain. In addition to this hypothesized inability to recognize emotions, it is likely that many patients try actively to suppress, deny, or cover up the emotional pain relating to adverse earlier life experiences. Rather than allowing themselves to experience this painful affect, they try to escape temporarily and avoid it through hard work and excessive activity or substance use (Blumer, 1982). After developing a chronic-pain problem, they become very inactive, preoccupied with pain, and consider themselves as having a "medical basis" for demanding pain-reduction drugs. At this point depression is frequently acknowledged, but only as a response to their unremitting pain.

The hypothesis that depression in a "masked" form precedes the development of chronic pain is controversial. Empirical evidence in support of this idea is lacking (Romano & Turner, 1985). Nevertheless, many features of this pattern do correspond with our clinical observations of some patients. Although Blumer and Heilbronn (1982) suggest that it applies to all patients with pain of uncertain etiology, we agree with Romano and Turner (1985) that it more likely applies to a subgroup of such patients.

Another hypothesis relating depression and pain is that both are the result of common neurobiological mechanisms. The fact that both pain and depression can respond to tricyclic antidepressants has been offered as support for neurochemical models (Butler, 1984; Feinmann, 1985). Centrally acting neuroregulators such as serotonin, dopamine, norepinephrine, and the endorphins have been mentioned as possible mediators (Ward et al., 1982). Sternbach (1976) suggested that chronic pain depletes brain serotonin. Since it is thought that serotonin is involved in both pain inhibition and depression, it is possible that depletion of this neurotransmitter underlies both pain and depression. More recently, Ward (1986) presented evidence for a serotonergic mechanism underlying the effectiveness of antidepressants in treating pain and depression. Specifically, those patients who responded positively to fenfluramine, a selective serotonin releaser, were also more likely to respond to tricyclic antidepressants. This supports the hypothesis that serotonin depletion underlies chronic pain and depression. Nevertheless, the precise role that serotonin and other neurochemicals play in chronic pain is far from clear (Feinmann, 1985).

Both the masked depression and neurochemical hypotheses may appear to be in opposition to cognitive and behavioral views that tend to view depression as a common psychological reaction to a chronic disabling physical condition such as chronic pain. Behavioral views are based on the idea that chronic-pain patients suffer a significant reduction in positive reinforcement (Fordyce, 1976). Rudy et al. (1988) and Kerns and Haythornthwaite (1988) present self-report questionnaire data that argue for a cognitive mediating model between pain and depression. According to the cognitive model there is not a direct and necessary relationship between pain and depression. Rather, cognitive mediating factors, such as perceptions of self-control and personal mastery, are important in determining depression. Thus, patients who view their pain as resulting in loss of personal control and as interfering with their life activities are more likely to be depressed.

Although we agree with the behavioral and cognitive perspectives, we do not see the various models relating pain and depression as being mutually exclusive or in opposition. Common biochemical mechanisms may underlie pain and depression for some people. Thus, antidepressant medications may alleviate both pain and depression in some individuals or reduce one complaint and not the other in other individuals. They may also have no effect on either pain or depression. More important in terms of the present discussion is our impression that some patients, as a result of early life experiences, have dispositional tendencies toward both depression and pain. Underlying depression and pain is the tendency to regard traumatic life events as beyond their personal control. Furthermore, such patients tacitly assume that their only recourse is to inhibit and suppress thoughts and feelings related to these events. The development of a chronic-pain condition becomes a partial solution. On the one hand, it confirms their basic belief that negative life events are uncontrollable. On the other hand, chronic pain does provide them with an acceptable target toward which they can channel their distress and openly express negative emotions.

Treatment

The question must be raised whether self-management training is sufficient to treat individuals whose chronic-pain syndromes have been preceded by a history of disturbed family relationships, emotional traumas, depression, and substance abuse. Although depression and substance abuse are addressed in self-management training, the therapeutic focus is primarily on the emotional and behavioral consequences of a chronic-pain syndrome. We believe that some of these individuals require more intensive psychotherapeutic approaches to address traumatic experiences or emotional disorders that preceded the chronic pain. Some professionals automatically assume that these patients are poor candidates for traditional psychotherapy (Blumer, 1982); we disagree. Roy (1982) has recommended dynamic psychotherapy for those who fit Engel's (1959) description of the pain-prone patient. In addition to psychodynamic approaches, it is our experience that many individuals can benefit from cognitive therapy for depression using the techniques developed by Beck and his colleagues (Beck et al., 1979). More complex structural and constructivist cognitive theories regarding the developmental origins of depression are also of value (Guidano & Liotti, 1983; Guidano, 1987).

In addition to cognitive approaches, we have used psychotherapeutic strategies involving emotional catharsis. Our approach differs from the one initially suggested by Beutler et al. (1986), who recommended use of Gestalt approaches to evoke negative emotions, especially anger. Although a recent study indicated that Gestalt therapy did result in decreased depression, it was no more effective than a control group condition that involved provision of information about the physiological bases of pain and the relationship of pain to daily events (Beutler et al., 1988). In contrast to contrived emotional evocation, we believe that ultimately it may be necessary for some patients to face their earlier painful experiences. The following case illustrates this.

E.G. was a 37-year-old divorced male with an 8-year history of chronic low back and left leg pain. He had undergone three unsuccessful back operations as well as psychiatric hospitalizations for depression and suicide attempts. When admitted to the pain program, he was unemployed, narcotic-dependent, and very depressed. During the course of treatment, it became apparent that he had come from a highly disturbed family background. As a youth, he had engaged in many antisocial activities. He also had had a long history of alcohol and drug abuse, unstable employment, and conflicted interpersonal relationships. After completing the pain program, he was seen for about 10 months of weekly individual psychotherapy. During therapy we focused on his early family experiences that had included, beginning at age 10, incestuous relations with both parents and an older brother. He eventually discovered that the older brother was actually his biological father. The relationships among these early experiences, patterns of social maladjustment, depression and guilt, and negative self-image were explored. Initially, E.G. found it extremely difficult to discuss his shameful past. However, as therapy progressed, his depression and substance abuse diminished, and he became reemployed. He also developed a new relationship with a women with whom he was able to discuss his shameful past. Pain complaints diminished entirely, even though he had made no use of the specific pain-coping strategies taught during self-management training.

Although not all cases are resolved this successfully, we have worked with several other patients whose pain was virtually eliminated during the course of psychotherapy. An important point to consider in these cases is that during therapy, pain management was not discussed at all. Sessions focused on early life experiences, their emotional consequences, and the relationship between these experiences and later adjustment. Considerable emphasis was placed on the development of a safe, trusting therapeutic relationship. As their earlier traumatic experiences were explored, it became readily apparent that these patients had never been able or allowed to express their emotions. For example, in the case cited above, the patient had experienced intensely conflicted emotions. In response to paternal and fraternal sexual abuse, he experienced a combination of rage, guilt, and enjoyment. Rage stemmed from the betrayal of parental trust and repeated violations of his psychosexual integrity. Guilt resulted from his perceptions that these occurrences must in some way have been his fault. At the same time, receiving physical affection and sexual gratification were experienced as pleasurable. The result of this conflict and confusion was repression of all feelings.

Rather than teaching these patients how to escape negative feelings through use of various cognitive reappraisal and coping strategies, we allow and even encouraged them to experience the painful affect associated with earlier experiences. This psychotherapeutic approach is essentially the cathartic method developed by Breuer and Freud (1895/1966) in their treatment of hysterical symptoms. Sometimes simply talking about these experiences in a therapeutic context is sufficient to evoke repressed, affectively charged memories. We have also utilized hypnotically induced age regression or just instructions to close the eyes and imagine reliving the specific painful experiences. This is especially indicated either for patients who have difficulty recalling the traumatic episodes or for those who can recall but have totally blocked off the associated affect.

It is important that patients be adequately prepared for these evocative approaches. Patients are warned that on an emotional level it can be a very painful process and that they may even experience a temporary increase in depression or somatic pain. They are told that this process is akin to lancing a painful boil, whereby it is necessary to experience increased pain in order to allow real healing to take place. Therapists also must be emotionally prepared, since it can be exceedingly unpleasant to be present as patients reexperience their painful past. Fortunately, however, as they are able to face their underlying sadness, guilt, anger, rage, feelings of parental abandonment and betrayal, and other traumatic experiences, we often find that their current symptoms gradually improve. Although emotional catharsis may in itself have benefit, we try to help these patients gain insight into the relationship between these past experiences and their more recent problems. Considerable attention is also given to helping them work on current problem issues and concerns using self-management approaches discussed in Chapter 7.

Some of these patients may also benefit from concurrent use of antidepressant medications, especially the tricyclics. A number of studies have reported positive benefits from these drugs with some pain patients (Aronoff et al., 1986; Butler, 1984). It is our observation that most patients do not respond very well when antidepressants are used as the sole or primary treatment.

The process of confronting traumatic events has received renewed attention in a series of studies by Pennebaker and his colleagues (Pennebaker, 1985; Pennebaker & Beall, 1986; Pennebaker, Hughes, & O'Heeron, 1987; Pennebaker, Kiecolt-Glaser, & Glaser, 1988). This line of research has suggested that the process of inhibiting or disclosing significant life experiences can have important implications on physical health. Specifically, these studies have shown that discussing or even just writing about thoughts and feelings associated with upsetting (traumatic) events can result in lower subjective distress, decreased utilization of medical services, and a potentially positive effect on measures of immune function. These beneficial effects may be viewed from two perspectives according to Pennebaker et al. (1988). First, they may result because the person no longer needs to engage in the stressful process of actively inhibiting or holding back his or her thoughts and feelings from others. Second, the process of facing a traumatic event may enable the person more readily to assimilate, reframe, or find meaning in the event. Although we are aware of no data regarding the beneficial effects of disclosure of such events on chronic pain, it may be hypothesized that a link does exist, especially among those who have previously inhibited or actively held back discussing traumatic events. According to Pennebaker et al. (1987), this process of inhibition can be physiologically stressful and eventually may result in adverse psychosomatic consequences.

PAIN AS A SOLUTION

Another type of patient who may respond poorly to self-management training is one who unconsciously utilizes pain complaints and disability as a solution to other life problems. Perhaps the most dramatic form of this phenomenon is found among those whose pain appears to be a hysterical conversion reaction. These patients usually have pain of sudden onset that enables them to escape or avoid an aversive or conflictive situation. In this sense, pain is a solution to a problem. Descriptions of pain may contradict known neuroanatomical facts and may be accompanied by relatively little emotional distress. Such patients are seldom referred to chronic-pain management programs.

Certain individuals fit the classic description of operant pain syndromes in that pain behavior is used to elicit environmental reinforcers. However, rather than simply having problems reinforced *after* the development of a pain condition, it appears that many of these individuals had *preexisting* problems. It is within this context that pain behavior is now used to elicit reinforcement that ameliorates the original problem. Consider, for example, the patient whose pain results in attention and nurturance from significant others. Whether or not these consequences are reinforcing and result in excessive pain behavior depends on the patient's history and personality factors before onset of the pain condition. Although most people have needs for attention and occasional nurturance, they do not require a disabling pain condition to have these needs met. Some report that attention and nurturance from family and friends in response to pain is annoying. Patients whose pain is maintained by social reinforcement often have a history of denying their dependence on others. As children they may have been ignored, abused, or excessively punished by their parents. Consequently, they develop strong needs to be loved and cared for. These needs must be denied and repressed, for to acknowledge them would be to risk further disappointment. The person may also try to compensate by striving to be independent and totally self-sufficient. It is against this background that ordinary social responses to an acute injury or illness episode can assume such reinforcing value. The person now has a justifiable reason for having dependency needs met. In short, pain has become a solution to what may have been a hidden life-long problem.

Although the past cannot be changed, it is possible to alter the current social consequences of pain behavior. This is the value of behavioral-management programs. Patients such as those just described can be given contingent social attention and recognition for more healthy behavior and for making the most of their lives in spite of a painful condition. Nevertheless, behavioral contingency management programs are only successful if the patient is willing to participate, relevant environmental reinforcers can be modified, and generalization can occur to the natural environment. Most behavioral and cognitive–behavioral self-management programs attempt to admit only those patients who express a willingness and desire to participate. However, as is seen in every chronic-pain program, there are some patients who meet the screening criteria, are admitted to the program, and then proceed to sabotage treatment every step of the way.

One common example of the individual who disrupts treatment is the patient who utilizes pain to maintain a pattern of substance dependency. Although such patients often profess a strong desire to learn more effective ways to manage their pain, they seem to go through the program half-heartedly and, on completion, report no benefit. It appears as though their "hidden agenda" was to fail the program in order to justify their need for drugs. In many of these patients, we find a history of substance abuse preceding the pain problem along with a tendency to deny that substance use is a problem.

For example, F.H. had a history of heavy marijuana use and alcohol abuse prior to dependence on large doses of narcotics to cope with chronic pain. He informed us that since he had discontinued marijuana and alcohol use on his own, he could not have been addicted. F.H. further asserted that his current need for narcotics was not caused by addiction but was necessary because his pain was so excruciating that nothing else worked. When confronted about what he really wanted from the pain program, he requested that we write a statement to his physician indicating that he should be given a stable amount of narcotics since alternative approaches were ineffective. This patient, in effect, needed his pain to justify his drug dependence.

As mentioned in Chapter 5, some individuals use chronic pain as a "self-handicapping" mechanism (e.g., "If it weren't for my disabling pain condition, I could have done . . . or, I could have been . . ."). In other words, chronic pain is used to justify failure to oneself or others. Without pain they would be expected to accomplish goals that they have not been able to reach. The following case illustrates this point.

G.I. was a 52-year-old married man with a 19-year history of chronic neck, shoulder, back, and leg pain following an automobile accident. Prior to his injury, G.I. had managed a small construction company that he had taken over from his father. Although he appeared to be very knowledgeable about the construction business, he had sold the company and lived off the proceeds before applying for disability compensation. During the prior 15 years, G.I. had spent much of his time searching for various cures, all to no avail. While participating in the pain program, he repeatedly informed other patients and staff how successful he could have been if it had not been for his accident. He also complained that the disability compensation system was not giving him anywhere near the support that he deserved. When confronted by staff and other patients about using his knowledge to return to some form of employment, he stated in no uncertain terms that he was far too disabled to work. During individual counseling sessions, it was discovered that as the oldest child he had been expected by his family to take over the father's company and make a great success of it. According to G.I.'s wife, when he initially took over the company, he suffered some financial setbacks, and his father was very critical about the way he was managing things.

It appeared to us that this patient in a sense needed his disabling pain condition to justify his failure to succeed vocationally. Therefore, the pain helped to keep his self-esteem intact.

We have encountered many other individuals for whom chronic pain appears to be a solution to preexisting personal or family problems. This usually occurs outside of the patient's awareness. If confronted with this observation, the patient will strongly deny that this is the case. Although some patients appear refractory to any form of pain treatment, it should not automatically be assumed that all patients in this category are inappropriate for self-management training. Some are able to learn alternative, more effective ways of coping with life problems without relying on their pain and disability.

PAIN AS A SOLUTION TO FAMILY PROBLEMS

It has been suggested that a person's physical health may be affected by disruptive events and dysfunctional interactional patterns within the family (Meissner, 1966, 1974; Weakland, 1977). These processes and events may be associated with the initiation or exacerbation of physical symptoms. Although the hypothesis that dysfunctional family processes play a causal role in physical health is controversial, there is general agreement that physical illness can have a disruptive effect on the family. A biopsychosocial model would predict that there are reciprocal interrelationships among a person's physical health and illness behavior, family interaction patterns, and stressful events within the family. Thus, it can be predicted that family factors interact with chronic-pain conditions as well.

It is known that chronic pain can have a negative impact on the patient's family (Ahern & Follick, 1985; Dura & Beck, 1988; Rowat & Knafl, 1985; Turk, Flor, & Rudy, 1987). More important in the present context is the observation that family members, especially the spouse, can help maintain and perpetuate a pain problem (Kremer, Sieber, & Atkinson, 1985; Payne & Norfleet, 1986). In addition to spousal reinforcement of pain behavior, it has been suggested that a couple may actually be invested in maintaining the pain (Delvey & Hopkins, 1982; Roy, 1985; Waring, 1977, 1982). Family systems theorists such as Haley (1963) and Minuchin (Minuchin, Rossman, & Baker, 1978) have noted that illness in a family member can serve to maintain homeostasis in a dysfunctional marriage or family system (cf. Grolnick, 1972). For example, the existence of pain may enable a couple to avoid confronting other problems that might threaten the stability of the marriage. The following is an example:

H.J. and his wife were both in their late 40s. Although H.J. had completed the pain-management program, he showed no improvement in his pain and disability behavior. Prior to developing a low back pain condition, he had worked as a shipping clerk, although his wife held a much more responsible, high-paying position in a large company. When they were first seen as a couple, H.J. appeared quite passive, and his wife frequently answered questions regarding his condition. It was eventually discovered that prior to the pain problem, H.J.'s wife had been very distressed over her inability to bear children. The wife also admitted fears that her husband, whom she considered very physically attractive, would leave her for another woman. The patient actually appeared to have been quite dependent and insecure regarding his masculine role identity and marriage to a woman who was obviously brighter and more competent than he. With the development of H.J.'s chronic-pain condition, it appeared that they had both found a solution. He was permitted to assume a more dependent role and no longer compete with his wife or cope in the world of adult responsibilities. She was able to meet her maternal needs by caring for her husband while at the same time feeling more secure that he would not leave her.

We have also noted, in support of suggestions by Waring (1982), that pain can sometimes serve as a substitute for intimacy in a marriage. This can occur when one or both partners have difficulty expressing or communicating their needs for affection and nurturance from the other. When pain serves an important role in stabilizing and maintaining a marital system, the chances of successful pain-management training are diminished. Some are also resistant to marital or family counseling, perhaps because it is too threatening. Others are much more amenable to such counseling. Consequently, when these marital or family-systems issues become apparent in pain-program sessions, the patient is usually referred for marital or family counseling after completing the program.

CHOOSING APPROPRIATE TREATMENT STRATEGIES

We have reviewed some examples of chronic-pain patients who may not respond well to self-management training programs. Rather than viewing this as a failure of self-management, we believe that such individuals were not well suited for such programs in the first place. In particular, we have suggested that for some individuals traditional psychotherapeutic approaches including individual, marital, and family psychotherapy may be more appropriate. We are aware that this suggestion is subject to criticism from those who adopt a more empirical, research orientation. In an important review of psychological approaches to chronic back pain, Turk and Flor (1984) appear to dismiss psychoanalytic and family-systems theories and the treatments they generate. Such approaches often utilize vague and ill-defined constructs and are largely based on anecdotal case evidence involving retrospective patient reports rather than well-controlled research investigations. Although we agree with these criticisms, we believe that family systems and psychodynamic therapeutic approaches can have a role in chronic-pain management *for selected patients*, even though such approaches lack the empirical support that is found with more cognitive and behavioral approaches. We do not necessarily subscribe to some of the vague constructs associated with structural family therapy (Minuchin, 1974) or psychoanalytic theory. Nevertheless, family systems approaches and individual psychotherapy that emphasize insight into developmental antecedents should be considered for those who do not respond or are not appropriate for cognitive–behavioral self-management training. For example, the problem-centered family-systems therapy model discussed by Roy (1986) should be considered even though no outcome studies exist which might support it. We also believe that the research perspective has its limitations, and that its value can be over-stated. We examine this issue in the next section.

Clinical versus Research Perspectives

In reviewing the chronic-pain treatment literature, one can find two general perspectives. Actually, these two perspectives can be found in the clinical and research literature concerning the treatment of most health problems. The clinical perspective emerges from the treatment imperative that physicians and other health care professionals have always assumed when confronted with an ill patient. Something must be done to help the patient. Relying on the wisdom of the day, the clinician's knowledge and experience, and sometimes little more than hunch, a particular course of treatment is chosen. In spite of the ancient dictum to do no harm, healers have always felt pressured to administer some kind of remedy to relieve pain and suffering. Consequently, just about every form of pain treatment imaginable has been tried, with some patients showing improvement, some showing no change, and others getting worse. In addition to experimenting with various treatments, clinicians also tend to devise theories explaining why their particular treatments work or do not work. Of course, these post hoc explanatory hypotheses are not necessarily valid.

The important point regarding the clinical perspective is that the choice of treatment techniques and their presumed theoretical bases may have little to do with available scientific research evidence. If clinicians were to utilize only those methods that rest on a strong empirical foundation, they would be extremely limited in what they could offer. When faced with those who present persistent pain complaints, the treatment imperative may predispose health care practitioners into trying various measures on a trial-and-error basis without any clear rationale why such measures should work. For example, consider the use of electrical stimulation in treating pain. These approaches, including surface stimulation (i.e., TENS) and invasive procedures (e.g., dorsal column stimulation), were first tried without any idea whether they would be effective or how they might be effective. When treatments such as these are successful, current pain theories such as gate-control mechanisms or endorphin production are invoked. Why these techniques close the spinal gate or increase endorphin production in one patient and fail to do so in another is never clear.

Sometimes a particular treatment technique is discovered serendipitously. It was discovered by accident that antidepressant medications, specifically tricyclics, can alleviate pain apart from their effects on depression. Biochemical hypotheses were later developed to explain these effects. Nevertheless, it is still not clear why a particular drug at a particular dosage has a positive effect on one patient's neurochemistry and no effect on another's. Ultimately, however, from the clinical perspective, what matters most is whether the patient who is being treated improves.

The research perspective is much more cautious and conservative than the clinical one. It emphasizes the discovery of scientific knowledge or truth. The fact that a particular treatment leads to improvement in a particular group of pain patients does not prove anything. It is known that pain is very responsive to the placebo effect. Controlled research with large enough samples, adequate comparison groups, and long enough follow-up is necessary to prove that a treatment technique is efficacious. This perspective also tends to be critical of post hoc theories that attempt to provide a rationale for the use of a particular technique. Theories must be stated in terms of testable hypotheses with their constructs operationalized and empirically tested before they can be considered valid.

Critical reviews of various topics within the chronic-pain literature usually lean toward the research perspective and offer methodological critiques (e.g., Flor & Turk, 1984; Turk & Flor, 1984). Reports based on anecdotal case information are given less weight than those based on control group comparison studies. Self-report data or patient's retrospective accounts are considered less valid than studies based on direct observation. The lack of supporting research and contradictory findings among studies are noted. Alternative explanations for treatment effects are offered. Reviews almost inevitably conclude that more research is needed before firm conclusions can be drawn.

Yet it should be apparent that clinical and research perspectives are both important and should complement one another. When faced with the difficult challenge of treating chronic-pain patients, clinicians usually feel obligated to "do something," irrespective of the presence or absence of strong research support for their methods. Nevertheless, treatment techniques should be evaluated through control-group outcome studies and adequate follow-up. The treatment imperative can sometimes lead clinicians in to trying unnecessary and even potentially harmful procedures. For example, it has been suggested that surgical treatment for low back pain is often based more on the patient's distress and illness behavior than it is on the presence of an actual physical disorder (Waddell, 1987). As noted by Fordyce (1988), clinicians often fail to distinguish between pain and suffering. Research that approaches pain from a biopsychosocial perspective can contribute significantly to identifying more effective interventions for particular patients.

One significant limitation faced by researchers when evaluating a particular treatment technique or etiological hypothesis is the tendency to look for firm conclusions that can apply to chronic-pain patients in general. This is often referred to as the "patient uniformity myth." Even when one limits consideration to a particular pain group such as headache patients or back pain patients, it is often forgotten that these are not homogeneous groups. Consequently, it makes no sense to search for the true etiology of chronic pain or the most effective treatment technique. A biopsychosocial systems model suggests that multiple interactive factors can result in a chronic-pain condition or chronic-pain syndrome. In other words, two individuals can present the same symptomatic complaints (e.g., chronic low back pain) and demonstrate essentially the same behavioral characteristics of the chronic-pain syndrome for very different reasons. For one individual the syndrome may have developed after the pain problem began, whereas for another, the syndrome may be symptomatic of life-long characterological problems. Furthermore, factors that initiated the chronic-pain condition may be quite different from those that are maintaining it. Facing researchers is the fact that whereas the biopsychosocial systems model has considerable appeal from a conceptual standpoint, it is difficult to test empirically, since it means taking into account multiple interacting dimensions.

As clinicians reading the chronic-pain literature, we find it very difficult to accept assertions that a particular etiological perspective applies to all of our patients let alone a specific treatment approach. At this point, we believe it is necessary to remain open to multiple perspectives and treatment approaches. In our experience, the self-management approach, as discussed in this book, is useful for a large number of chronic-pain patients because it is flexible and relevant to several different types of chronic-pain patients. It is also well suited for inpatient or outpatient group programs. Nevertheless, we do not expect every patient to benefit from each component in the same way. For example, some appear to benefit primarily from training in cognitive pain/stress-coping skills, others benefit primarily from physical reconditioning exercises and reinforcement for increased activity level, and still others are helped through withdrawal of narcotic analgesics. Research perspectives, on the other hand, usually approach multicomponent programs by asking which single component or set of components is necessary or most efficacious. Dismantling or sequential mantling research designs are then recommended. From our perspective, the value of component analysis is often overstated since it fails to recognize the heterogeneity of chronic-pain patients.

In spite of our belief in the flexibility of self-management training, we have pointed out that this approach is not for everyone. We believe that a greater effort should be made to identify particular treatment strategies or programs that are most relevant for a particular pain patient rather than make all patients fit a particular treatment approach. There are presently no clear or agreed-upon guidelines that can help pain treatment practitioners determine which approach is more suitable for which patient. We agree with those who believe that matching patients and treatments should be given more of a research priority (Malone & Strube, 1988; Turk & Flor, 1984). From their meta-analysis of nonmedical treatments for chronic pain, Malone and Strube (1988) conclude, "the critical issue at this time is not demonstration of the superiority of one type of treatment over others, but instead the identification of the type of treatment most likely to provide long-term benefit from a specific type of pain for a specific type of patient" (p. 237).

Presently, from a clinical perspective, efforts to identify the most appropriate treatment for a patient depends primarily on adequate assessment. The challenge of assessment is that it be thorough enough to identify those factors (biological, psychological, or social) that are most responsible for maintaining pain in a particular patient. The identification of these factors will then determine the recommended course of treatment. If treatment fails to address the most significant contributing factors, it is more likely to fail. Unfortunately, it is often very difficult to assess accurately some of the most important psychological contributing factors, since most pain patients tend to deny their relevance. Although many patients will admit that their pain causes cognitive, emotional, behavioral, and social problems, many others are completely unaware of factors that are maintaining their pain.

We believe that in addition to the use of psychological tests, clinicians must rely heavily on behavioral observation and thorough history taking. Although the common self-report test instruments used with pain patients have the advantage of being standardized and easy to administer, they often miss some of the more subtle factors associated with pain. For example, family influences on pain are particularly difficult to ascertain via questionnaires (Flor, Turk, & Rudy, 1987). Even more difficult to obtain through standard questionnaires is in-depth information about the patient's family of origin. Sensitive clinicians will often find important clues from the patient's history, from information obtained from spouses, and by observing the patient's interactions with others. Such an assessment focus will aid in more accurate identification of relevant psychosocial contributing factors. In particular, it is important to determine the extent to which these factors played a role prior to or subsequent to the development of chronic pain.

Rather than attempting to place all chronic-pain patients in to a single rigid treatment category and then dismissing those who do not fit, pain-treatment professionals should recognize that no single clinical approach nor any one professional discipline has all the answers. We can identify at least four general treatment models for chronic-pain conditions that we label as medical, self-management, psychotherapeutic, and supportive counseling models. Each model is appropriate for some but not all chronic-pain patients.

Medical Management

The medical model is the preferred approach when the primary factors contributing to ongoing pain are more clearly biological (e.g., an ongoing disease process), and the patient is coping as well as can be expected. Because of the chronic nature of the underlying disorder, treatment is usually conservative and focused on symptom management. Patients who appropriately fit this model have generally learned to accept their pain condition as a fact of life and are no longer intent on finding total pain relief or a medical cure. In spite of chronic pain, they are able to minimize its disabling effects and lead reasonably satisfying and fulfilling lives. These patients are not generally depressed, they do not depend on narcotics to cope with pain, and they do not use pain behavior for its reinforcing consequences. Most have healthy social relationships, are relatively active, and have learned to live within their physical limitations. Since they do not repeatedly seek medical solutions, these individuals are usually not referred to multimodal chronic-pain management programs. Because of the circumscribed nature of their pain condition, they may benefit from more focused treatment approaches such as trigger point injections, physical therapy procedures, biofeedback training, and hypnosis.

Self-Management

The second category applies to those who have developed many features of the chronic-pain syndrome such as narcotic dependence, preoccupation with pain and other somatic complaints, sleep disturbance, inactivity, physical deconditioning, social withdrawal, low self-esteem, depression, and repetitive efforts to seek medical cures in spite of many prior failed attempts. Some have clear medical indications of injury or disease, and others do not. Often they had managed their lives reasonably well prior to onset of their pain condition. Thereafter, they seem to have been caught in a downward spiral revolving around chronic pain and disability. Some individuals with long histories of chronic pain were able to effectively self-manage their pain for a number of years and then, as their situation changed, began the downward spiral. For example, we have treated a number of individuals who had satisfactorily coped with chronic back pain for over 30 years. During most of their adult life they fit more into the first category. However, as they became older, developed new health problems, retired from active employment, and suffered various losses and disappointments, they began turning more and more to the health care system and gradually developed many features of the chronic-pain syndrome. These individuals are all appropriate candidates for a comprehensive self-management treatment program as discussed in this book. This type of program is primarily educational in that new coping skills are taught, maladaptive pain behaviors are not rewarded, and previously learned adaptive behaviors are encouraged and positively reinforced. When treatment is successful, these individuals learn to cope with their pain in a manner that is essentially the same as those in the first category who have learned to do so without any special pain management training.

Psychotherapeutic Management

The third category of patient primarily requires a psychotherapeutic treatment model. These patients also typically possess many features of the chronic-pain syndrome found among those in the second category. However, unlike those in the second category, these individuals have a long history of significant psychosocial and characterological problems preceding onset of their chronic pain. More often then not, these problems have gone untreated by mental health professionals. Depression, problems with intimate relationships, and substance abuse commonly preceded their chronic pain. In addition to overt psychiatric symptoms, many of these individuals have diagnosable personality disorders such as dependent, passive–aggressive, and histrionic personalities (Fishbain, Goldberg, Meagher, Steele, & Rosomoff, 1986). Individuals in this category are less likely to respond well to self-management training. Preexisting problems are readily apparent in an initial evaluation. Alternatives to a formal chronic-pain management program can then be explored, such as treatment for substance abuse, antidepressant medication, marital or family therapy, and more intensive individual psychotherapy. Others for whom it is not readily apparent may first be unsuccessfully treated with medical and self-management approaches before it is discovered that other psychosocial problems predominate. They can then be offered various psychotherapeutic approaches including individual or family therapy.

When first considering such patients for psychotherapy, it is important not to dismiss pain complaints as irrelevant. Pain complaints can be responded to with medication and instruction in self-management techniques, and at the same time the focus can be shifted to relevant psychosocial issues. Since most of these individuals are not "psychologically minded" and have no prior experience with psychotherapy, it is often useful to begin with more structured approaches including cognitive and behavioral methods. With some patients who are initially reluctant to interact with a psychologist, we may begin with biofeedback training and then, as a trusting therapeutic relationship develops, gradually shift discussion to other more sensitive issues. As therapy proceeds, the therapist focuses more on developmental themes as they relate to current problems. The dynamics of the therapeutic relationship may also be used to illuminate the patient's habitual ways of responding to significant others. Throughout this process, the therapist should remain relatively active while continuing to place responsibility for change onto the patient.

Supportive Counseling

Finally, there are those patients whose pain complaints seem to follow a personal crisis or significant life change perceived as disruptive. Such crises may result from loss of a significant relationship on which the patient was highly dependent. Another common precipitant is a change in roles that threaten basic identity such as loss of employment, retirement, or growth and departure of children from the home. Prior to their pain complaints, these individuals functioned reasonably well in that they had never sought psychological assistance or shown signs of significant psychopathology as is the case for those in the third category. Medical evaluations usually fail to identify factors that would adequately account for the degree of pain complaints. Depending on the length of time following onset of pain complaints these patients may or may not possess features of the chronic-pain syndrome. Rather than requiring a comprehensive pain management program or intensive psychotherapy, most of these individuals can benefit from short-term supportive counseling or crisis intervention. Visits to primary health care providers with complaints of pain or other somatic symptoms occur because the person is psychologically unsophisticated or too ashamed to seek psychological assistance. Once the real problems are addressed, complaints of pain usually cease.

It should not be forgotten that the vast majority of patients in each of these four categories present honest complaints of somatic pain. Little will be accomplished by dismissing the pain complaints of those who present obvious psychological problems. The biopsychosocial systems model also applies to patients in each category. Irrespective of the primary etiology, physiological, cognitive, emotional, behavioral, and environmental factors all interact even though the pattern of interaction may be markedly different across patients.

Clinicians should beware of professional biases that may lead them to focus on some factors (e.g., medical versus psychological) and ignore others. Even among those psychiatrists and psychologists who emphasize the role of psychological factors, there are often clear indications of bias. In particular, there is a tendency for some to assume that psychological factors always result from the pain problem, whereas others assume that all psychological problems existed prior to onset of the pain condition. Those in the former group lean toward a self-management, pain-coping treatment model utilizing cognitive–behavioral approaches (e.g., Blanchard & Andrasik, 1985; Philips, 1988; Turk et al., 1983), whereas those in the latter group emphasize more of a psychiatric treatment model involving medication and/or insight-oriented psychodynamic psychotherapy (e.g., Blumer & Heilbronn, 1982; Pilowsky & Bassett, 1982).

Additionally, those who emphasize self-management are much less concerned whether or not "objective" medical findings exist for a particular patient, whereas those who emphasize preexisting psychiatric conditions assume that this applies only to those with minimal evidence for organic etiology. Although it is obvious that our bias is toward self-management, we believe it is important that each group recognize the contributions of the other. One reason for including this chapter is to acknowledge that some chronic-pain patients do have significant preexisting psychiatric conditions that should be addressed with more conventional psychotherapeutic approaches as opposed to cognitive–behavioral/educational approaches.

Since no single professional discipline can encompass all aspects of chronic pain, clinicians must be willing to seek consultation and advice from other specialties. Recognition of this fact has led to the tremendous growth in multidisciplinary pain clinics. Irrespective of which discipline is involved in evaluating a particular chronic-pain patient, we believe that if a comprehensive biopsychosocial model is kept in mind, it is much more likely that appropriate treatment strategies will be utilized.

IMPLICATIONS OF THE BIOPSYCHOSOCIAL MODEL AND SELF-MANAGEMENT

In conclusion, we would like to mention the fact that the biopsychosocial model and self-management are relevant to far more than chronic-pain patients. During the past 10 years or so there has been growing application of this model and self-management treatment approaches to patients with a variety of chronic disease conditions including asthma, diabetes, certain gastrointestinal disorders, hypertension, Raynaud's disease, and various neurological and neuromuscular conditions (Holroyd & Creer, 1986). In spite of many well-publicized advances, technologically oriented biomedicine has been generally less successful in the management of chronic illness. This lack of success is particularly important in that 8 of the 10 most common causes of death in the United States are chronic diseases, including the three leading causes of death—heart disease, cancer, and cerebrovascular diseases (Burish & Bradley, 1983).

From our perspective, the primary implication of the biopsychosocial model for chronic disease is the fact that it places greater responsibility on the individual rather than the health care system. The willingness to assume personal responsibility lies at the essence of our definition of self-management. Personal responsibility can be seen in two areas. First, and probably most important, is prevention of injury and disease (Stachnik, Stoffelmayr, & Hoppe, 1983). Prevention is based on the recognition that lifestyle factors play a significant role in the etiology of most chronic diseases. In an important article on personal responsibility, John Knowles (1977) points out:

> Prevention of disease means forsaking the bad habits which many people enjoy—overeating, too much drinking, taking pills, staying up at night, engaging in promiscuous sex, driving too fast, and smoking cigarettes— or, put another way, it means doing things which require special effort— exercising regularly, going to the dentist, practicing contraception, ensuring harmonious family life, submitting to screening examinations. (p. 59)

Elsewhere, he states,

> Central to the culture is faith in progress through science, technology, and industrial growth; increasingly peripheral to it is the idea, vis-à-vis health, that over 99% of us are born healthy and made sick as a result of personal misbehavior and environmental conditions. The solution to the problems of ill health in modern American society involves individual responsibility, in the first instance, and social responsibility through public legislative and private voluntary efforts, in the second instance . . . Meanwhile, the people have been led to believe that national health insurance, more doctors, and greater use of high-cost, hospital-based technologies will improve health. Unfortunately, none of them will. (pp. 58-60)

Prevention has considerable relevance to chronic pain as well. It is likely that many painful injuries could be prevented by following better safety practices. These include on-the-job injuries, injuries occurring at home, and sports-related injuries. Back injuries, in particular, can be prevented by utilization of proper body mechanics, maintenance of a healthy body weight, and maintenance of the spine and its supporting structures through regular physical exercise. Prevention is also necessary to keep painful acute conditions from turning into chronic-pain syndromes.

The second area of personal responsibility is the day-to-day management of the chronic physical condition. Here the patient's goal is to prevent the development of secondary problems that make the original condition worse. Compliance with medical treatment procedures and recommendations, the adoption of a healthy, balanced lifestyle, and the development and utilization of healthy social supports may accomplish much in this direction.

In addition to delivering quality medical care, physicians have other important responsibilities when treating those with chronic diseases. First, greater attention should be given to the development of a collaborative working relationship with chronically ill patients (Hanson, 1986). In contrast to authoritarian and patronizing approaches, a collaborative relationship is based on mutual respect and shared responsibility for the development of a treatment program. Second, it is important that the limits of technological medicine be recognized and communicated to patients. Although physicians and other health care professionals can be valuable resources, it is ultimately the responsibility of the chronically ill person to adopt a healthy behavioral lifestyle, establish good coping resources such as social supports, and utilize cognitive coping methods that facilitate the most healthy and rewarding life possible in spite of chronic pain or other disease conditions.

References

Adler, R.H., Zlot, S., Hurny, C., & Minder, C. (1989). Engel's "psychogenic pain and the pain-prone patient": A retrospective, controlled clinical study. *Psychosomatic Medicine, 51*, 87–101.

Ahern, D.K., & Follick, M.J. (1985). Distress in spouses of chronic pain patients. *International Journal of Family Therapy, 7*, 247–257.

Alberti, R., & Emmons, M.L. (1982). *Your perfect right*. San Louis Obispo, CA: Impact Publishing.

American Academy of Orthopaedic Surgeons. (1965). *Joint motion: Method of measuring and recording*. Chicago: Author.

Andrasik, F., & Holroyd, K.A. (1980). A test of specific and nonspecific effects in the biofeedback treatment of tension headache. *Journal of Consulting and Clinical Psychology, 48*, 575–586.

Aronoff, G.M., & Wagner, J.M. (1987). The pain center: Development, structure and dynamics. In G.D. Burrows, D. Elton, & S.V. Gordon (Eds.), *Handbook of chronic pain management* (pp. 407–424). Amsterdam: Elsevier.

Aronoff, G.M., Wagner, J.M., & Spangler, A.S. (1986). Chemical interventions for pain. *Journal of Consulting and Clinical Psychology, 54*, 769–775.

Atkinson, J.H., Slator, M.A., Grant, I., Patterson, T.L., & Garfin, S.R. (1988). Depressed mood in chronic low back pain: Relationship with stressful life events. *Pain, 35*, 47–55.

Barber, J. (1982). Incorporating hypnosis in the management of chronic pain. In J. Barber & C. Adrian (Eds.), *Psychological approaches to the management of pain* (pp. 40–59). New York: Brunner/Mazel.

Barber, J. (1986). Hypnotic analgesia. In A.D. Holzman & D.C. Turk (Eds.), *Pain management: A handbook of psychological treatment approaches* (pp. 151–167). New York: Pergamon Press.

Barlow, D.H. (1988). *Anxiety and its disorders: The nature and treatment of anxiety and panic*. New York: Guilford Press.

Beck, A.T. (1976). *Cognitive therapy and the emotional disorders*. New York: International Universities Press.

Beck, A.T. (1978). *Depression inventory*. Philadelphia: Center for Cognitive Therapy.

Beck, A.T., Rush, A.J., Shaw, B.F., & Emery, G. (1979). *Cognitive therapy of depression*. New York: Guilford Press.

Beecher, H.K. (1955). The powerful placebo. *Journal of the American Medical Association, 159,* 1602–1606.

Belar, C.D., & Kibrick, S.A. (1986). Biofeedback in the treatment of chronic back pain. In A.D. Holzman & D.C. Turk (Eds.), *Pain management: A handbook of psychological treatment approaches* (pp. 131–150). New York: Pergamon Press.

Benson, H. (1975). *The relaxation response*. New York: William Morrow.

Bernstein, D.A., & Borkovec, T.D. (1973). *Progressive relaxation training: A manual for the helping professions*. Champaign, IL: Research Press.

Bernstein, D.A., & Given, B.A. (1984). Progressive relaxation: Abbreviated methods. In R.L. Woolfolk & P.M. Lehrer (Eds.), *Principles and practice of stress management* (pp. 43–69). New York: Guilford Press.

Beutler, L.E., Engle, D., Oro'-Beutler, M.E., Daldrup, R., & Meredith, K. (1986). Inability to express intense affect: A common link between depression and pain? *Journal of Consulting and Clinical Psychology, 54,* 752–759.

Beutler, L. E., Daldrup, R., Engle, P., Guest, P., Corbishley, A., & Meredith, K.E. (1988). Family dynamics and emotional expression among patients with chronic pain and depression. *Pain, 32,* 65–72.

Blanchard, E.B., & Andrasik, F. (1985). *Management of chronic headaches: A psychological approach*. New York: Pergamon Press.

Blumer, D. (1982). Psychiatric aspects of chronic pain: Nature, identification and treatment of the pain-prone disorder. In R.H. Rothman & F.A. Simeone (Eds.), *The spine* (Vol. 2, pp. 1090–1117). Philadelphia: W.B. Saunders.

Blumer, D., & Heilbronn, M. (1982). Chronic pain as a variant of depressive disease: The pain-prone disorder. *Journal of Nervous and Mental Disease, 170,* 381–406.

Bortz, W.M. (1984). The disuse syndrome. *Western Journal of Medicine, 141,* 691–694.

Brena, S.F., & Hammonds, W.D. (1983). Nerve blocks: Chemical and deep stimulation analgesia. In S.F. Brena & S.L. Chapman (Eds.), *Management of patients with chronic pain* (pp. 195–203). New York: SP Medical & Scientific Books.

Bresler, D. (1979). *Free yourself from pain*. New York: Simon & Schuster.

Breuer, J., & Freud, S. (1966). *Studies on hysteria*. New York: Avon. (Originally published in 1895)

Budzynski, T.H., Stoyva, J.M., Adler, C.S., & Mullaney, D.J. (1973). EMG biofeedback and tension headache: A controlled outcome study. *Seminars in Psychiatry, 5,* 397–410.

Burish, T.G., & Bradley, L.A. (1983). Coping with chronic disease: Definitions and issues. In T.G. Burish & L.A. Bradley (Eds.), *Coping with chronic disease: Research and applications* (pp. 3–12). New York: Academic Press.

Burns, D.D. (1980). *Feeling good: The new mood therapy*. New York: William Morrow.

Butler, S. (1984). Present status of tricyclic antidepressants in chronic pain therapy. In C. Benedetti, C.R. Chapman, & G. Moricca (Eds.), *Advances in pain research and therapy, Vol. 7* (pp. 173–197). New York: Raven Press.

Clelland, J., Savinar, E., & Shepard, K. (1987). The role of the physical therapist in chronic pain management. In G.D. Burrows, D. Elton, & G.V. Stanley (Eds.) *Handbook of chronic pain management*, (pp. 243–258). Amsterdam: Elsevier.

Copp, L.A. (1987). The role of the nurse in chronic pain management. In G.D. Burrows, D. Elton, & G.V. Stanley (Eds.), *Handbook of chronic pain management*, (pp. 227–242). Amsterdam: Elsevier.

Crelin, E.S. (1973). A scientific test of chiropractic theory. *American Scientist, 61,* 574–580.

Crisson, J.E., & Keefe, F.J. (1988). The relationship of locus of control to pain coping strategies and psychological distress in chronic pain patients. *Pain, 35,* 147–154.

Crue, B.L. (1983). The peripheralist and centralist views of chronic pain. *Seminars in Neurology, 3,* 331–339.

Crue, B.L., & Pinsky, J.J. (1984). An approach to chronic pain of non-malignant origin. *Postgraduate Medical Journal, 60,* 858–864.

Daniels, L., & Worthingham, C. (1986). *Muscle testing: Techniques of manual examination* (5th ed.). Philadelphia: W.B. Saunders.

Delvey, J., & Hopkins, L. (1982). Pain patients and their partners: The role of collusion in chronic pain. *Journal of Marital and Family Therapy, January,* 135–142.

Deyo, R.A., Diehl, A.K., & Rosenthal, M. (1986). How many days of bed rest for acute low back pain? A randomized clinical trial. *New England Journal of Medicine, 315,* 1064–1070.

DiMatteo, M.R., & DiNicola, D.D. (1982). *Achieving patient compliance: The psychology of the medical practitioner's role.* New York: Pergamon Press.

Dishman, R.K. (1982). Compliance/adherence in health-related exercise. *Health Psychology, 1,* 237–267.

Dolce, J.J., & Raczynski, J.M. (1985). Neuromuscular activity and electromyography in painful backs: Psychological and biomechanical models in assessment and treatment. *Psychological Bulletin, 97,* 502–520.

Doliber, C. (1984). Role of the physical therapist at pain treatment centers. *Physical Therapist, 64,* 905–909.

Doran, D.M.L., & Newell, D.J. (1975). Manipulation in treatment of low back pain: A multicenter study. *British Medical Journal, 2,* 161–164.

Dura, J.R., & Beck, S.J. (1988). A comparison of family functioning when mothers have chronic pain. *Pain, 35,* 70–89.

D'Zurilla, T.J. (1986). *Problem-solving therapy: A social competence approach to clinical intervention.* New York: Springer.

D'Zurilla, T.J., & Goldfried, M.R. (1971). Problem solving and behavior modification. *Journal of Abnormal Psychology, 78,* 107–126.

Eisenberg, L. (1977). Disease and illness: Distinctions between profession and popular ideas of sickness. *Cultural Medicine and Psychiatry, 1,* 9–23.

Ellis, A. (1982). *Reason and emotion in psychotherapy.* New York: Lyle Stuart.

Ellis, A., & Harper, R. (1975). *A new guide to rational living* (2nd ed.). Hollywood, CA: Wilshire Books.

Engel, G.L. (1959). "Psychogenic" pain and the pain-prone patient. *American Journal of Medicine, 26,* 899–918.

Engel, G.L. (1977). The need for a new medical model: A challenge for biomedicine. *Science, 196,* 129–136.

Erickson, M.H. (1982). The interspersal hypnotic technique for symptom correction and pain control. In J. Barber & C. Adrian (Eds.), *Psychological approaches to the management of pain* (pp. 100–117). New York: Brunner/Mazel.

Evans, F.J. (1981). The placebo response in pain control. *Psychopharmacology Bulletin, 17,* 72–76.

Feinmann, C. (1985). Pain relief by antidepressants: Possible modes of action. *Pain, 23,* 1–8.

Fernandez, E. (1986). A classification system of cognitive coping strategies for pain. *Pain, 26,* 141–151.

Fishbain, D.A., Goldberg, M., Meagher, B.R., Steele, R., & Rosomoff, H. (1986). Male and female chronic pain patients categorized by DSM-III diagnostic criteria. *Pain, 26,* 181–197.

Flor, H., & Turk, D.C. (1984). Etiological theories and treatments for chronic back pain. I. Somatic models and interventions. *Pain, 19,* 105–121.

Flor, H., Turk, D.C., & Rudy, T.E. (1987). Pain and families. II. Assessment and treatment. *Pain, 30,* 29–45.

Fordyce, W.E. (1976). *Behavioral methods for chronic pain and illness.* St. Louis: C.V. Mosby.

Fordyce, W.E. (1988). Pain and suffering: A reappraisal. *American Psychologist, 43,* 276–283.

France, R.D., & Krishnan, K.R.R. (1985). The dexamethasone suppression test as a biological marker of depression in chronic pain. *Pain, 21,* 49–55.

Frymoyer, J.W. (1988). Back pain and sciatica. *New England Journal of Medicine, 318,* 291–300.

Gerber, K.E., & Nehemkis, A.M. (Eds.). (1986). *Compliance: The dilemma of the chronically ill.* New York: Springer.

Gildenberg, P.L., & DeVaul, R.A. (1985). *The chronic pain patient: Evaluation and management.* Basel: S. Karger.

Goldstine, M. (Ed.). (1975). *The research status of spinal manipulative therapy, HEW Publication No. 76.* Bethesda: U.S. Government Printing Office.

Gore, D.R., Sepic, S.B., Gardner, G.M., & Murray, M.P. (1987). Neck pain: A long-term follow-up of 205 patients. *Spine, 12,* 1–5.

Grolnick, L.A. (1972). Family perspective of psychosomatic factors in illness: A review of the literature. *Family Process, 11,* 457–486.

Guidano, V.F. (1987). *Complexity of the self: A developmental approach to psychopathology and therapy.* New York: Guilford Press.

Guidano, V.F., & Liotti, G. (1983). *Cognitive processes and emotional disorders.* New York: Guilford Press.

Haley, J. (1963). Marriage therapy. *Archives of General Psychiatry, 8,* 213–234.

Hanson, R.W. (1986). Physician–patient communication and compliance. In K.E. Gerber & A.M. Nehemkis (Eds.), *Compliance: The dilemma of the chronically ill* (pp. 182–212). New York: Springer.

Heide, F.J., & Borkovec, T.D. (1983). Relaxation-induced anxiety: Paradoxical anxiety enhancement due to relaxation training. *Journal of Consulting and Clinical Psychology*, *51*, 171–182.

Hojnacki, L.H., & Halfman-Franey, M. (1985). *Handbook of cardiac rehabilitation for nurses and other health professionals*. Reston, VA: Reston Publishing Co.

Holroyd, K.A., & Creer, T.L. (Eds.). (1986). *Self-management of chronic disease*. New York: Academic Press.

Holroyd, K.A., Penzien, D.B., Hursey, K.G., Tobin, D.L., Rogers, L., Holm, J.E., Marcille, R.J., Hall, J.R., & Chila, A.G. (1984). Change mechanisms in EMG biofeedback training: Cognitive changes underlying improvements in tension headache. *Journal of Consulting and Clinical Psychology*, *52*, 1039–1053.

Holzman, A.D., Rudy, T.E., Gerber, K.E., Turk, D.C., Sanders, S.H., Zimmerman, J., & Kerns, R.D. (1985). Chronic pain: A multiple-setting comparison of patient characteristics. *Journal of Behavioral Medicine*, *8*, 411–422.

Illich, I. (1976). *Medical nemesis*. New York: Pantheon Books.

Jones, N.L., & Campbell, E.J.M. (1982). *Clinical exercise testing* (2nd ed.). Philadelphia: W.B. Saunders.

Kane, R.L., Olsen, D., Leymaster, D., Woolley, F.R., & Fisher, F.D. (1974). Manipulating the patient: A comparison of the effectiveness of physician and chiropractor care. *Lancet*, *1*, 1333–1336.

Keel, P.J. (1984). Psychosocial criteria for patient selection: Review of studies and concepts for understanding chronic back pain. *Neurosurgery*, *15*, 935–941.

Kendall, F.P. (1983). *Muscles: Testing and function* (3rd ed). Baltimore: Williams & Wilkins.

Kerns, R.D., & Haythornthwaite, J.A. (1988). Depression among chronic pain patients: Cognitive–behavioral analysis and effect on rehabilitation outcome. *Journal of Consulting and Clinical Psychology*, *56*, 870–876.

Kerns, R.D., Turk, D.C., & Rudy, T.E. (1985). The West Haven–Yale Multidimensional Pain Inventory (WHYMPI). *Pain*, *23*, 345–356.

Knowles, J.H. (1977). The responsibility of the individual. In J.H. Knowles (Ed.), *Doing better and feeling worse: Health in the United States* (pp. 57–80). New York: W.W. Norton.

Knox, V.J. (1973). Cognitive strategies for coping with pain: Ignoring vs. acknowledging. *Dissertation Abstracts International*, *34 (5-B)*, 2308.

Kremer, E.F., Sieber, W., & Atkinson, J.H. (1985). Spousal perpetuation of chronic pain behavior. *International Journal of Family Therapy*, *7*, 258–270.

Kroger, W.S., & Fezler, W.D. (1976). *Hypnosis and behavior modification: Imagery condition*. Philadelphia: J.B. Lippincott.

Lazarus, A., & Fay, A. (1975). *I can if I want to*. New York: Warner Books.

Lazarus, R.S., & Folkman, S. (1984). *Stress, appraisal, and coping*. New York: Springer.

Leventhal, H., & Everhart, D. (1979). Emotion, pain, and physical illness. In C.E. Izard (Ed.), *Emotions in personality and psychopathology* (pp. 263–299). New York: Plenum Press.

Leventhal, H., Meyer, D., & Narenz, D. (1980). The common sense representation of illness danger. In S. Rachman (Ed.), *Medical psychology* (Vol. 2, pp. 7–30). New York: Pergamon Press.

Leventhal, H., & Narenz, D. (1983). A model for stress research with some implications for the control of stress disorders. In D. Meichenbaum & M.E. Jaremko (Eds.), *Stress reduction and prevention* (pp. 5–38). New York: Plenum Press.

Leventhal, H., Zimmerman, R., & Gutmann, M. (1984). Compliance: A self-regulation perspective. In W.D. Gentry (Ed.), *Handbook of behavioral medicine* (pp. 369–436). New York: Guilford Press.

Loeser, J.D. (1982). Concepts of pain. In M. Stanton-Hicks & R. Boas (Eds.), *Chronic low back pain* (pp. 145–148). New York: Raven Press.

Loeser, J.D. (1985). Pain due to nerve injury. *Spine, 10,* 232–235.

Long, D.M. (1983). A peripheralist view of chronic pain: Observations in transcutaneous electrical stimulation. *Seminars in Neurology, 3,* 341–346.

Long, D.M., Filtzer, D.L., BenDebba, M., & Hendler, N.H. (1988). Clinical features of the failed back syndrome. *Journal of Neurosurgery, 69,* 61–71.

Malone, M.D., & Strube, M.J. (1988). Meta-analysis of non-medical treatments for chronic pain. *Pain, 34,* 231–244.

Marlatt, G.A. (1985). Lifestyle modification. In G.A. Marlatt & J.R. Gordon (Eds.), *Relapse prevention* (pp. 280–348). New York: Guilford Press.

Marlatt, G.A., & Gordon, J.R. (1985). *Relapse prevention.* New York: Guilford Press.

Mason, L.J. (1980). *Guide to stress reduction.* Culver City, CA: Peace Press.

McCaffery, M. (1979). *Nursing management of the patient with pain* (2nd ed.). Philadelphia: J.B. Lippincott.

McCaul, K.D., & Malott, J.M. (1984). Distraction and coping with pain. *Psychological Bulletin, 95,* 516–533.

McGuigan, F.J. (1984). Progressive relaxation: Origins, principles, and clinical applications. In R.L. Woolfolk & P.M. Lehrer (Eds.), *Principles and practice of stress management* (pp. 12–42). New York: Guilford Press.

McKay, M., Davis, M., & Fanning, P. (1981). *Thoughts and feelings: The art of cognitive stress intervention.* Richmond, CA: New Harbinger.

Mechanic, D. (1962). The concept of illness behavior. *Journal of Chronic Diseases, 15,* 189–194.

Mechanic, D. (1978). *Medical sociology* (2nd ed.). New York: Free Press.

Meichenbaum, D. (1977). *Cognitive–behavior modification: An integrative approach.* New York: Plenum Press.

Meichenbaum, D., & Turk, D.C. (1987). *Facilitating treatment adherence: A practitioner's guidebook.* New York: Plenum.

Meissner, W.W. (1966). Family dynamics and psychosomatic processes. *Family Process, 5,* 142–161.

Meissner, W.W. (1974). Family process and psychosomatic disease. *International Journal of Psychiatry in Medicine, 5,* 411–430.

Melzack, R., & Casey, K.L. (1968). Sensory, motivational, and central control determinants of pain: A new conceptual model. In D. Kenshalo (Ed.), *The skin senses* (pp. 423–443). Springfield, IL: Charles C. Thomas.

Melzack, R., & Perry, C. (1975). Self-regulation of pain: The use of alpha-feedback and hypnotic training for the control of chronic pain. *Experimental Neurology, 46,* 452–469.

Melzack, R., & Perry, C. (1980). *Psychological control of pain.* New York: B M A Audio Cassettes.

Melzack, R., & Torgerson, W.S. (1971). On the language of pain. *Anesthesiology, 34,* 50–59.

Melzack, R., & Wall, P.D. (1965). Pain mechanisms: A new theory. *Science, 150,* 971–979.

Melzack, R., & Wall, P.D. (1982). *The challenge of pain.* New York: Basic Books.

Mendelson, G., Selwood, T.S., Kranz, H., Loh, T.S., Kidson, M.A., & Scott, D.S. (1983). Acupuncture treatment of chronic back pain: A double-blind placebo-controlled trial. *American Journal of Medicine, 74,* 49–55.

Miller, A. (1984). *For your own good: Hidden cruelty in child-rearing and the roots of violence.* New York: Farrar, Straus, & Giroux.

Miller, J.G. (1978). *Living systems.* New York: McGraw-Hill.

Miller, S.M. (1979). Controllability and human stress: Method, evidence and theory. *Behaviour Research and Therapy, 17,* 287–304.

Minuchin, S. (1974). *Families and family therapy.* Cambridge, MA: Harvard University Press.

Minuchin, S., Rossman, B., & Baker, L. (1978). *Psychosomatic families: Anorexia nervosa in context.* Cambridge, MA: Harvard University Press.

Morse, R.H. (1983). Toward an eclectic stance in algology. *Seminars in Neurology, 3,* 355–358.

Nachemson, A. (1979). A critical look at treatment for low back pain. *Scandinavian Journal of Rehabilitation Medicine, 11,* 143–147.

Olshan, N.H. (1980). *Power over your pain without drugs.* New York: Rawson, Wade Publishers.

Osterweis, M., Kleinman, A., & Mechanic, D. (Eds.). (1987). *Pain and disability: Clinical, behavioral, and public policy perspectives.* Washington, DC: National Academy Press.

Parsons, T. (1958). Definitions of health and illness in the light of American values and social structure. In E.G. Jaco (Ed.), *Patients, physicians and illness* (pp. 165–187). New York: Free Press.

Payer, L. (1988). *Medicine and culture.* New York: Henry Holt.

Payne, B., & Norfleet, M.A. (1986). Chronic pain and the family: A review. *Pain, 26,* 1–22.

Pennebaker, J.W. (1982). *The psychology of physical symptoms.* New York: Springer-Verlag.

Pennebaker, J.W. (1985). Traumatic experience and psychosomatic disease: Exploring the roles of behavioral inhibition, obsession, and confiding. *Canadian Psychology, 26,* 82–95.

Pennebaker, J.W., & Beall, S. (1986). Confronting a traumatic event: Toward an understanding of inhibition and disease. *Journal of Abnormal Psychology, 95,* 274–281.

Pennebaker, J.W., Hughes, C., & O'Heeron, R.C. (1987). The psychophysiology of confession: Linking inhibitory and psychosomatic processes. *Journal of Personality and Social Psychology, 52*, 781–793.

Pennebaker, J.W., Kiecolt-Glaser, J.K., & Glaser, R. (1988). Disclosure of traumas and immune function: Health implications for psychotherapy. *Journal of Consulting and Clinical Psychology, 56*, 239–245.

Philips, H.C. (1988). *The psychological management of chronic pain: A treatment manual.* New York: Springer.

Pilowsky, I., & Bassett, D. (1982). Individual dynamic psychotherapy for chronic pain. In R. Roy & E. Tunks (Eds.), *Chronic pain: Psychosocial factors in rehabilitation* (pp. 107–125). Baltimore: Williams & Wilkins.

Poppen, R. (1988). *Behavioral relaxation training and assessment.* New York: Pergamon Press.

Reynolds, D.K. (1976). *Morita psychotherapy.* Berkeley: University of California Press.

Reynolds, D.K. (1984). *Constructive living.* Honolulu: University of Hawaii Press.

Roberts, A.H. (1986). The operant approach to the management of pain and excess disability. In A.D. Holzman & D.C. Turk (Eds.), *Pain management: A handbook of psychological treatment approaches* (pp. 10–30). New York: Pergamon Press.

Romano, J.M., & Turner, J.A. (1985). Chronic pain and depression: Does the evidence support a relationship? *Psychological Bulletin, 97*, 18–34.

Rowat, K.M., & Knafl, K.A. (1985). Living with chronic pain: The spouse's perspective. *Pain, 23*, 259–271.

Roy, R. (1982). Pain-prone patient: A revisit. *Psychotherapy and Psychosomatics, 37*, 202–213.

Roy, R. (1985). The interactional perspective of pain behaviour in marriage. *International Journal of Family Therapy, 7*, 271–283.

Roy, R. (1986). A problem-centered family systems approach in treating chronic pain. In A.D. Holzman & D.C. Turk (Eds.), *Pain management: A handbook of psychological treatment approaches* (pp. 113–130). New York: Pergamon Press.

Rudy, T.E., Kerns, R.D., & Turk, D.C. (1988). Chronic pain and depression: Toward a cognitive–behavioral mediation model. *Pain, 35*, 129–140.

Rudy, T.E., Turk, D.C., & Brena, S.F. (1988). Differential utility of medical procedures in the assessment of chronic pain patients. *Pain, 34*, 53–60.

Sacerdote, P. (1982). Techniques of hypnotic intervention with pain patients. In J. Barber & C. Adrian (Eds.), *Psychological approaches to the management of pain* (pp. 60–83). New York: Brunner/Mazel.

Sachs, L.B., Feuerstein, M., & Vitale, J.H. (1977). Hypnotic self-regulation of chronic pain. *American Journal of Clinical Hypnosis, 20*, 106–113.

Sarno, J.E. (1984a). *Mind over back pain.* New York: William Morrow.

Sarno, J.E. (1984b). Therapeutic exercise for back pain. In J.V. Basmajian (Ed.), *Therapeutic exercise* (4th ed., pp. 441–463). Baltimore: Williams & Wilkins.

Schultz, J.H., & Luthe, W. (1969). *Autogenic therapy, Vol. I: Autogenic Methods.* New York: Grune & Stratton.

Schwartz, G.E. (1980). Behavioral medicine and systems theory: A new synthesis. *National Forum, 60*, 25–30.

Shapiro, A.K., & Morris, L.A. (1978). Placebo effects in medical and psychological therapies. In S.L. Garfield & A.E. Bergin (Eds.), *Handbook of psychotherapy and behavior change* (2nd ed., pp. 369–410). New York: John Wiley.

Shapiro, D. H. (1980). *Meditation: Self-regulation strategy and altered state of consciousness*. New York: Aldine.

Shealy, C.N. (1977). *90 Days to self-health*. New York: Dial Press.

Sifneos, P. (1973). The prevalence of "alexithymic" characteristics in psychosomatic patients. *Psychotherapy and Psychosomatics, 22*, 255–262.

Soskis, D.A. (1986). *Teaching self-hypnosis*. New York: W.W. Norton.

Spiro, H.M. (1986). *Doctors, patients and placebos*. New Haven: Yale University Press.

Spitzer, W.O., & Quebec Task Force on Spinal Disorders. (1987). Scientific approach to the assessment and management of activity-related spinal disorders: A monograph for clinicians. *Spine, 12* (Suppl.), S1–S59.

Stachnik, T., Stoffelmayr, B., & Hoppe, R.B. (1983). Prevention, behavior change, and chronic disease. In T.G. Burish & L.A. Bradley (Eds.), *Coping with chronic disease: Research and applications* (pp. 447–473). New York: Academic Press.

Sternbach, R.A. (1974). *Pain patients: Traits and treatment*. New York: Academic Press.

Sternbach, R.A. (1976). The need for an animal model of pain. *Pain, 2*, 2–4.

Sternbach, R.A. (1987). *Mastering pain: A twelve-step program for coping with chronic pain*. New York: G.P. Putnam's Sons.

Stone, G.C. (1979). Health and the health system: A historical overview and conceptual framework. In G.C. Stone, F. Cohen, & N.E. Adler (Eds.), *Health psychology* (pp. 1–18). San Francisco: Jossey-Bass.

Stroebel, C.F. (1983). *QR: The quieting reflex*. New York: Berkley Books.

Tan, S.Y. (1982). Cognitive and cognitive–behavioral methods for pain control: A selective review. *Pain, 12*, 201–228.

Taylor, H., & Curran, N. (1985). *The Nuprin pain report*. New York: Louis Harris & Associates.

Temoshok, L. (1983). Emotion, adaptation, and disease: A multidimensional theory. In L. Temoshok, C. Van Dyke, & L.S. Zegans (Eds.), *Emotions in health and illness: Theoretical and research foundations* (pp. 207–233). New York: Grune & Stratton.

Turk, D.C., & Flor, H. (1984). Etiological theories and treatments for chronic back pain. II. Psychological models and interventions. *Pain, 19*, 209–233.

Turk, D.C., Flor, H., & Rudy, T.E. (1987). Pain and families. I. Etiology, maintenance and psychosocial impact. *Pain, 30*, 3–27.

Turk, D.C., Meichenbaum, D., & Genest, M. (1983). *Pain and behavioral medicine: A cognitive–behavioral perspective*. New York: Guilford Press.

Turk, D.C., & Rudy, T.E. (1987). Towards a comprehensive assessment of chronic pain patients. *Behaviour Research and Therapy, 25*, 237–249.

Turk, D.C., & Rudy, T.E. (1988). Toward an empirically derived taxonomy of chronic pain patients: Integration of psychological assessment data. *Journal of Consulting and Clinical Psychology, 56*, 233–238.

Turner, J.A., & Chapman, C.R. (1982). Psychological interventions for chronic pain: A critical review. I. Relaxation training and biofeedback. *Pain*, *12*, 1–21.

Valkenburg, H.D., & Haanen, H.C.M. (1982). The epidemiology of low back pain. In A.A. White & S.L. Gordon (Eds.), *Symposium on ideopathic low back pain* (pp. 9–22). St. Louis: C.V. Mosby.

Violon, A. (1982). The process involved in becoming a chronic pain patient. In R. Roy & E. Tunks (Eds.), *Chronic pain: Psychosocial factors in rehabilitation* (pp. 20–35). Baltimore: Williams & Wilkins.

von Bertalanffy, L. (1968). *General systems theory*. New York: Braziller.

Wachtel, P.L. (Ed.). (1982). *Resistance: Psychodynamic and behavioral approaches*. New York: Plenum Press.

Waddell, G. (1987). A new clinical model for the treatment of low-back pain. *Spine*, *12*, 632–644.

Waddell, G., Kummel, E.G., Lotto, W.N., Graham, J.D., Hall, H., & McCulloch, J.A. (1979). Failed lumbar disc surgery and repeat surgery following industrial injuries. *Journal of Bone and Joint Surgery*, *61*, 201–206

Waddell, G., McCulloch, J.A., Kummel, E.G., & Venner, R.M. (1980). Nonorganic physical signs in low back pain. *Spine*, *5*, 117–125.

Waddell, G., Morris, E.W., DiPaola, M.P., Bircher, M., & Finlayson, D. (1986). A concept of illness tested as an improved basis for surgical decisions in low-back disorders. *Spine*, *11*, 712–719.

Ward, N.G. (1986). Tricyclic antidepressants for chronic low-back pain: Mechanisms of action and predictors of response. *Spine*, *11*, 661–665.

Ward, N.G., Bloom, V.L., Dworkin, S., Fawcett, J., Narasimhachari, N., & Friedel, R. (1982). Psychobiological markers in coexisting pain and depression: Toward a unified theory. *Journal of Clinical Psychiatry*, *43*, 32–38.

Waring, E. (1977). The role of the family in symptom selection and perpetuation in psychosomatic illness. *Psychotherapy and Psychosomatics*, *28*, 253–259.

Waring, E. (1982). Conjoining marital and family therapy. In R. Roy & E. Tunks (Eds.), *Chronic pain: Psychosocial factors in rehabilitation* (pp. 151–165). Baltimore: Williams & Wilkins.

Weakland, J.H. (1977). "Family somatics": A neglected edge. *Family Process*, *16*, 263–272.

Weber, H. (1983). Lumbar disc herniation: A controlled, prospective study with ten years of observation. *Spine*, *8*, 131–140.

White, A.A. (1983). *Your aching back: A doctors's guide to relief*. New York: Bantam Books.

Williams, R.C. (1988). Toward a set of reliable and valid measures for chronic pain assessment and outcome research. *Pain*, *35*, 239–251.

Wolff, H.G., & Wolf, S. (1958). *Pain*. Springfield, IL: Charles C. Thomas.

Zborowski, M. (1952). Cultural components in responses to pain. *Journal of Social Issues*, *8*, 16–30.

Zola, I.K. (1966). Culture and symptoms: An analysis of patients' presenting complaints. *American Sociological Review*, *31*, 615–630.

Index